Effective Communication
in Nursing

Effective Communication in Nursing
Theory and Practice

JOSEPH F. CECCIO, Ph.D.
Department of English
The University of Akron
Akron, Ohio

CATHY M. CECCIO, R.N., B.A.
Department of Nursing Education
Barberton Citizens Hospital
Barberton, Ohio

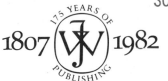

A WILEY MEDICAL PUBLICATION
JOHN WILEY & SONS
New York • Chichester • Brisbane • Toronto • Singapore

Library of Congress Cataloging in Publication Data:

Ceccio, Joseph F.

—Effective communication in nursing.
  (A Wiley medical publication)
  Includes bibliographies and index.
   1. Communication in nursing. 2. Nursing—
Authorship. I. Ceccio, Cathy M. II. Title.
III. Series. [DNLM: 1. Communication—Nursing
texts. 2. Writing—Nursing texts. WY 87 C388e]

RT23.C4   610.73'0141   81–15999
ISBN 0–471–07911–1   AACR2

Printed in the United States of America

10 9 8 7 6 5 4 3 2 1

For Tina, Linda, and Chris
J.F.C.

For Helen, Don, and Kate
C.M.C.

Preface

Written by a specialized writing teacher and a nursing staff development educator, *Effective Communication in Nursing: Theory and Practice* aims at (1) preparing professional nursing students to handle the many writing and speaking tasks they will encounter on the job and (2) helping people already working in the profession to communicate more effectively. One belief that underlies all the chapters of this textbook is that effective communication can be measured in terms of whether or not the sender's message has had the intended impact on its receivers.

To educate people in evaluating the results of their writing and speaking, this book presents learner-centered materials in ways designed to bridge the gap between abstractions in textbooks and the specific problems that confront professional nurses. In style, we try to practice what we teach about successful visual and verbal communication. Selection of content and coverage is based on the communication situations and problems nurses most frequently encounter. Chapters progress in order of increasing difficulty and complexity; the material within each chapter is also arranged in order of increasing difficulty. Each chapter contains a set of behavioral objectives at the outset and ends with a summary, exercises, references, and further readings.

We take a theory-and-practice approach to our subject. Basically, we view communication as adaptation and as the essence of nursing. In addition, the numerous exercises add up to a special feature of the book, for they are based on authentic situations and problems in nursing communication. Although we focus primarily on written communication, we also treat several important nonwritten modes of communication.

By surveying the communication process in nursing interactions, Chapter 1 provides the theoretical framework for the discussion of communication practice that follows. But theory also appears throughout the other seven chapters where appropriate.

Chapter 2 carefully discusses client-centered documentation within the nursing process; Chapter 3 treats writing readable health information for the client.

The fourth chapter covers documenting within the health care system.

Chapter 5 continues this discussion by exploring the topic of writing and the nurse leader.

In examining some key nonwritten modes of communication, the sixth chapter gives the book a wider focus than would be achieved if just written communication were dealt with.

Chapter 7 guides readers through researching and writing for publication, as it simultaneously supplies timely and helpful advice on a variety of related topics from literature review and journal selection to manuscript preparation and the editorial process.

Finally, the eighth chapter reviews communicating about employment in the profession, and the material there can help both new graduates and more experienced professional nurses with the communications aspect of getting a position or changing jobs.

Every attempt has been made to avoid using stereotyped language in this book; but sometimes, for the sake of simplicity and conciseness, *she* or *he* and the like appear alone.

The support and assistance of many colleagues and friends must certainly be acknowledged. We owe special thanks to Letetia H. Paulk, Vicky McGaffick, Marie Gayetsky, Carol Storad, and Grace Duncan, all of Barberton Citizens Hospital; to Frederik N. Smith and Claibourne E. Griffin, both of The University of Akron; to Rosa L. Weinert, of the Ohio State Board of Nursing; and to Cathy Somer, of Healthways Communications, Inc. We also wish to acknowledge, with thanks, that various forms appearing in this book were used with the kind permission of Barberton Citizens Hospital, M.A. Bernatovicz, Administrator. Many thanks are also due to the Wiley Medical Division staff, especially to Jim D. Simpson and Don Schott. Judith M. Major, of The University of Akron, was our excellent manuscript typist, and Lynne Chiles assisted in the typing. Vickie Slee, graphic designer, did the illustrations. Finally, we recognize each other's help, for this book was truly a joint effort—neither of us could have written it without the other.

J.F.C.
C.M.C.

Contents

CHAPTER 1

The
Communication Process
in Nursing Interactions

Objectives

After studying this chapter, you will be able to

1. List the four purposes of communication.
2. Define effective communication.
3. Explain the nature of the communication process.
4. Differentiate between the mathematical theory of communication and the behavioral theory of communication.
5. Define the components of the response-oriented communication model.
6. Identify seven barriers to effective communication.
7. Describe three communication facilitators.
8. Discuss the Roy adaptation model and its application to the communication process in nursing.

Effective communication in nursing is crucial because the essence of nursing is really communication. To a great extent, communication is *the* tool with which to accomplish collaborative patient care goals. The hallmark of a nursing professional is awareness of and the ability to use both formal and informal communication systems.

COMMUNICATION SITUATIONS

As our starting point, let's briefly consider various examples of nursing communications that take place during a single day in Charlestown, a representative North American community.

At Charlestown City Hospital, Brenda MacGregor, R.N., scans the bulletin board at the nurses' station on 4-West. While waiting for the change-of-shift team report to begin, she decides to read the notices that have accumulated in just the 2 weeks she was on vacation: the CCH pharmacy newsletter highlighting nursing implications for a potent antibiotic, a memo from the nursing office listing several job openings, the staff development calendar for the next month, a description of the new UCG procedure from the lab, and a notice from Dietary changing patients' tray times, among others. Did the notices do their job? Has Brenda missed anything?

Every day at 7 AM the nurses on different units give reports, and often the communication modes vary. On 3-South, for example, the nurses tape their reports. On 5-North they make walking rounds. On 6-South they meet in the examination room to give each other an oral report. Downstairs the clinical supervisors also meet face to face.

At work in another area, Henry Martin, associate director of surgical nursing at CCH, carefully reviews recent patient classification system reports to gather the information he needs to help determine staffing levels for the 3 PM to 11 PM shift. Three floors below, Helen Sloan, patient teaching coordinator, is planning a new health education booklet, "How to Care for Your Cast." Other pamphlets already completed in this series include "Questions and Answers About Diabetes," "Your Fractured Hip," and "Your New Hip." Helen tries to write to the appropriate audience and so consciously employs the *you* viewpoint, modern style, and a positive tone.

Mrs. Leonard bursts out of room 337, waves to the head nurse at the end of the corridor, points to her pocket, then extends her palm. The head nurse readily responds by carrying the soft-restraint key down the hall to Mrs. Leonard. A nonverbal message was sent, apparently received, and even acted upon. But was it the same message Mrs. Leonard had in mind? Has there been communication or miscommunication here?

Later in the morning Stephanie Baylor, senior primary nurse in the intensive care unit, interviews Mr. Clifford in the privacy of the family waiting room about his wife's previous health history. Mrs. Clifford was in an automobile accident yesterday, and her multiple injuries make it impossible for her to give the nurse much subjective data about her past health habits, lifestyle, or sensory-motor status. Stephanie will use the information she gathers from Mr. Clifford to write up a nursing history; data gathered from the nursing history, as well as systematic observations of Mrs. Clifford's physiological status, will enable Stephanie to formulate a nursing diagnosis and to initiate a plan of care to meet Mrs. Clifford's unique needs. When Stephanie is off duty, the care plan will serve as the major communication tool for all nurses about Mrs. Clifford's nursing care.

In her office, Anita Johnson, psychiatric clinical nurse consultant, puts the finishing touches on a special report. Her feasibility study on the potential for a 35-bed acute care psychiatric unit at CCH must be submitted by noon tomorrow. Shortly thereafter, the hospital administrator must decide whether to fund this unit or not, but clearly the quality of Anita's report will play a significant part in the decision-making process. It could even be *the* determining factor.

Meanwhile, from her home on Charlestown's west side, Jenny Howard types her letter of application and résumé for a staff nurse opening at a hospital 600 miles away. She needs to relocate with her husband, who is being transferred in 2 months. The documents she mails today could win her an interview (still another form of communication). Even as Jenny proofreads her materials, Ed Miller carefully completes his application form in the personnel department at Charlestown's Visiting Nurse Association. He will be interviewed within the next half-hour for a staff position as liaison caseworker with Charlestown-area hospitals.

Later, during this same day, still other nursing communication situations take place in Charlestown:

1. At a health maintenance organization, the pediatric nurse practitioner examines 6-year-old Billy for the third time in 4 months for an upper respiratory infection. She documents her findings, assessment, and plan of care in the problem-oriented format.
2. Across town at the University Student Health Center, three R.N.s begin a series of group counseling sessions on how to deal with stress. Final examinations start in 2 weeks.
3. The in-service education coordinator of Deerfield Manor, a 250-bed extended care facility, is developing a proposal for a series of programs for the professional nurses on the topic of concepts and skills in psychosocial assessment of the elderly. The proposal discusses the programs' objectives, content, length, and faculty.
4. At a downtown Planned Parenthood clinic, the senior family nurse practitioner needs to dictate a letter of justification for a new teaching videotape that demonstrates how to insert a diaphragm.
5. Even though the family nurse practitioner at the city-sponsored outpatient clinic attempts to reassure a young construction worker that because today's specimen shows no evidence of bacteria, his severe urinary tract infection has probably cleared up, the young patient still grows agitated and chain-smokes while waiting to see the part-time physician on duty. He must return to work today or be fired.

Back at CCH there are more communication problems as the day wears on. For one thing, rumor has it that Mrs. Kennedy, director of nurses, has suddenly decided to retire early. Rather than allow a feeling of uncertainty to continue too long, she schedules a late afternoon meeting for supervisors and head nurses so that she can explain how her health requires her to retire at the end of the month. In another development—just 30 minutes before Mrs. Kennedy's meeting—the chairperson of CCH's nursing education department learns that her request to hire two more R.N.s has been approved but that her request for more office space on the second floor has been denied. What will she be thinking about at Mrs. Kennedy's meeting?

Becky Watson's evening is busy, for five new patients have been admitted to the surgical unit and she must see to it that their nursing assessments are complete, to ensure effective care plans. In order to care for Mr. Cox in room 409, Becky uses a written care plan; in the Cardex she checks med cards; then she reads the physician's progress notes. At the same time two floors up, Chuck Blackwell, senior primary nurse, greets Mr. Livingston as he is brought to the unit. Chuck takes him to his room, introduces him to his roommate, and shows him which closet and drawers are his. Although he has never been in a hospital before, Mr. Livingston now feels less anxious about being here. So far, he feels he has been treated as an individual.

Each of these situations or examples involves communication—with the potential for miscommunication—in a nursing context. We have looked briefly at just a few instances of communication in practice on a single workday. But the need for communication is always present; the process is continual.

IMPORTANCE OF COMMUNICATION

Communication—in particular, *successful* communication—keeps organizations such as Charlestown City Hospital and the others just mentioned functioning efficiently, smoothly, even humanely. In addition, it plays a crucial part in your nursing career and in your personal life.

Meeting Organizational Goals

As the very lifeblood of an organization, effective communication helps a goal-directed group of people attain understanding, cooperation, and results. Early in his book *Communication and Interpersonal Relations* William V. Haney states:

> It is eminently clear that effective communication is essential in business, in governmental and military organizations, in hospitals, schools, communities, homes—anywhere that people deal with one another. It is difficult, in fact, to imagine any kind of interpersonal activity which does not depend upon communication in some form or other.[1]

Now, as you might expect, the higher up you go in an organization, the more time you will likely spend communicating. According to Haney, "aside from communicating—speaking, writing, listening, reading, and thinking (*intra*personal communication)—an organization's top administrator does virtually nothing!"[2] Today, many nurse professionals devote more time to these five communication activities than to actual nursing interventions, which can often be delegated to other members of the health care team.

Organizational communication activities may be categorized as internal or external. In a hospital, for example, job-related written and spoken communications that inquire, inform, or persuade may travel upward, downward, or laterally—yet still remain within the organization. On the other hand, communications designed especially for people outside the organization—a hospital's annual report, its instructional pamphlets, its telephone replies to former or potential clients—can also contribute positively or negatively to meeting organizational goals. Later, we will have more to say about the theory and practice of adapting to different audiences in nursing communication.

Satisfying Professional Responsibilities

Developing solid communication skills will help you secure a respectable entry-level nursing position, keep that position, and even win promotions. In his now classic article, "What Do You Mean I Can't Write?" John Fielden puts the ability to communicate at the top of the list of requisites for promotability:

1. Ability to communicate
2. Ambition—drive
3. College education
4. Ability to make sound decisions
5. Self-confidence
6. Good appearance
7. Ability to get things done with and through people
8. Capacity for hard work[3]

As a professional, you will need to continue your education after graduation in order to keep up with the ever-evolving field of nursing. And as a communicator interacting with both patients and other health professionals, you will also need to refine your written, oral, and nonverbal communication skills and techniques. Perhaps Eleanor C. Hein's description of therapeutic communication as "planning so that one consciously influences less able persons into directions and actions beneficial to their welfare"[4] pinpoints the need for, and the rewards of, studying effective communication in nursing.

Fulfilling Personal Roles

Although effective communication is vital to the life of the organization and is one key to a successful nursing career, it is also important in your personal life. Serious students of nursing communication often succeed better in their remaining nursing courses once they learn more about the theory and practice of communicating orally and in writing for the profession. Further, as an individual in society, you will constantly face off-the-job situations that require a letter, a report, a telephone call, or perhaps a speech as the appropriate solution. The benefits that you gain now from understanding and applying nursing communication principles can carry over to your present—and future—family, social, and community relationships.

PURPOSES OF COMMUNICATION

Before we discuss the process and problems of communication, we should pause for a moment to review the basic purposes of communication. Four communication objectives are

1. To inquire
2. To inform
3. To persuade
4. To entertain

If we keep these four specific applications in mind, the theoretical foundation for the study of effective communication in nursing that we are about to lay will make more sense.

Messages that inquire include direct, often simple requests for information, assistance, services, or supplies for which no special persuasive effort seems necessary to motivate the receiver of the message to action.

Messages that inform convey information—whether positive, neutral, or negative—to the intended audience. As you will see, strategies for handling good-news and neutral messages (in which the factual or subject content is stressed) differ from strategies for handling bad-news messages (in which the affective or feeling content is stressed).

Messages that persuade motivate the receiver to act or behave in a way that he or she may not have thought about before. When you anticipate unfavorable audience reaction to your special request for agreement or action, you will need to plan an indirect or inductive approach rather than simply a direct approach to the situation.

Messages that entertain tend to be mixed messages because they often include both informative and persuasive components. Their chief purposes are to divert, to amuse, to decrease tension, and sometimes to build rapport with the receiver. Whether such messages take a written, oral, or nonverbal form, they can be more significant for nurse communicators than is generally recognized.

WHAT EFFECTIVE COMMUNICATION IS

One obvious and rather oversimplified way of looking at communication is to define it as a static entity instead of as the vital process that it really is. Thus, you will encounter such definitions as "transmitting or imparting information, feelings, thoughts, messages" or "sharing information, ideas, attitudes, understanding." But these tell only part of the story, for they focus more on the sender of the message than on the receiver. One belief that underlies all the chapters of this text is that effective communication can be measured in terms of whether or not the sender's message has had the intended impact on its receiver.

When the receiver fails to understand precisely what the sender intended to convey, miscommunication results. And to complicate the picture further, not all communication is even intentional, for it is possible to communicate unintentionally as well. One head nurse we know habitually uses the stereotyped expression "And how are *we* this morning?" to greet each patient on the floor. Her words carry an obvious surface meaning, yet her word choice and tone of voice may also carry metacommunications, or meanings beyond those stated. One patient may resent the impersonal *we*; another may take offense at being addressed like a child. The head nurse's opening line does communicate although it is not fully effective in terms of its receivers.

Defining the word *communication* through still more words has its dangers and its limitations, to be sure. Yet, before attempting to develop our own working model of the communication process, we can at least isolate in the abstract some communication variables that we will soon study in operation. As a complex process, communication involves sending *and* receiving information, feelings, and attitudes—usually verbally but frequently nonverbally—that produce some *response,* hopefully a favorable one. In the *effective* communication, therefore, a message is transmitted and received, but real communication occurs only once the receiver provides some response to the sender through feedback, and the sender reacts to or otherwise acknowledges the response. Often, the sending of feedback does not come easily to the receiver, and feelings, emotions, and values may impede the success of the substantive message. Whenever the "feedback loop" is not completed (that is, the receiver does not send or the original sender does not react to or ignores the feedback message), the communication process breaks down. Thus, effective communication requires the observation of consistent feedback and demands commitment and perseverance on the part of the communicators.

In their 1973 article on therapeutic communication, David S. Fuller and Gustavo M. Quesada perceptively write:

> We propose that in the practice of *all* human therapeutics (including those of medicine and surgery, dentistry, nursing, speech

therapy, and others) the effectiveness of communication between the participants in the system is a major determinant of
whether that therapy succeeds. Success in therapy . . . refers appropriately to attaining not only the goals of the therapist but also
those of the patient.[5]

In other words, Fuller and Quesada believe that it is the proper use
of feedback in the communication process that ensures the success of
meaningful, therapeutic interaction. Only by sharing information
and giving each other feedback do the clinician and the patient reveal
their goals.

By learning more about the nature of communication in this chapter
and about its applications in nursing in subsequent chapters, you can
enhance your effectiveness and success as a professional nurse.

COMMUNICATION AS A PROCESS

Just within the last 30 years or so, research and writing in the field of
human communication theory and practice have dramatically increased,
both in quantity and in quality. And because communication is a genuinely interdisciplinary subject, human communication theory has incorporated significant contributions from such varied fields as psychology,
sociology, linguistics, anthropology, human relations, mass communication, philosophy, and information technology.

Before moving on to the discussion of selected communication theory
that follows, we first need to agree on the meaning of two essential concepts: (1) operational definition and (2) process. In order to avoid, as much
as possible, using words and more words to define words, we will look at
the communication process *in action,* that is, *operationally.* You should
try to picture a communication event involving two people (perhaps a
nurse and a client) in a face-to-face spoken exchange (although, with
some modifications, a written communication situation between people
would also work here). How does the communication process work and,
sometimes, how does it not work?

Second, we need to share a common meaning for the word *process.* Communication theorist David K. Berlo offers the following:

If we accept the concept of process, we view events and relationships as dynamic, on-going, ever-changing, continuous. When
we label something as a process, we also mean that it does not
have *a* beginning, *an* end, a fixed sequence of events. It is not
static, at rest. It is moving. The ingredients within a process interact; each affects all of the others.[6]

The frequently cited paradox that a person can never step in the same river twice, for the person is different and so is the river, illustrates well this concept of process. For purposes of analysis and discussion, we may temporarily "freeze" the communication process in order to describe its ingredients or elements. Yet we also recognize the limits of language, especially words printed on a page, for dealing with any process as complicated as communication.

Usefulness of Theories and Models

Theories are worthwhile when they assist us in realizing what we are doing so that we can do it even better. A carefully constructed theory may explain a specified set of phenomena or help us predict the future. Thus, a theory may be viewed as a set of interrelated concepts or abstractions that gives a systematic, logical view of a phenomenon or an event. But despite considerable progress in recent years, no single communication theory yet exists that is perfect or complete. In the words of Francis W. Weeks and Daphne A. Jameson, "We still do not have a theory that explains adequately what happens when some communications are successful and some are not."[7] For our purposes, however, knowing two important theories—the mathematical theory and the behavioral theory—will advance you toward your goal of becoming a better nurse communicator.

Models often accompany theories, and they can be valuable also. A model, which might appear visually as a diagram or verbally as an outline or a list, is a symbolic representation of an object, an event, a process, or a situation. A model may be said to represent the structure or abstraction of the theory, while theory can be defined as a set of scientific principles representing function. A good model can help you define a problem, discover a solution, and then measure that solution's success or failure; it can help you visualize the communication process, for example, so that you can understand it better. Communication models provide several other advantages that will become apparent shortly.

Mathematical Theory

Composed of two remarkable and rather technical papers on communication theory, one by Claude E. Shannon of Bell Telephone Laboratories and the other by Warren Weaver of The Rockefeller Foundation, *The Mathematical Theory of Communication* was published in 1949. Shannon investigated the technical or engineering problems of transmitting a message from sender to receiver. Weaver augmented Shannon's work in electronic communication by blending the engineering and the human applications of this theory. That device which, for better or worse, affects our lives so much today—the computer—is built upon a mathematical communication concept.

The Shannon-Weaver communication system consists of the following factors:

1. Information source (encoder)
2. Message
3. Transmitter
4. Signal
5. Channel
6. Noise source
7. Received signal
8. Receiver (decoder)
9. Message
10. Destination[8]

In order to visualize these factors in operation, consider one segment of a face-to-face spoken exchange between a nurse and an aide concerning the necessity of Mr. Baker's not having food or drink until after his blood sample has been drawn later this morning. Here the *information source,* or encoder, is the nurse's brain; the selected *message* consists of the soon-to-be-spoken words, "Be sure Mr. Baker has nothing to eat or drink this morning until after his blood sample is drawn." The *transmitter* is the nurse's voice box, which produces the varying sound pressure, the *signal,* which is transmitted through the air, the *channel.* Any unwanted additions, deletions, or distortions in the transmitted signal are called *noise.* Physical noise, such as the unplanned misuse or misunderstanding of words by either the sender or the receiver, could also alter the signal. Finally, the signal becomes the *received signal* when it reaches the *decoder* (in this case, the aide's ear). The *message as received* by the aide arrives at its *destination,* the listener's brain. Perhaps the message sent by the nurse is the same as the message received by the aide. But perhaps it is not.

Weaver discusses three types of communication problems. First, how accurately can the symbols of communication be transmitted? This is the technical problem. Second, how precisely do the transmitted symbols convey the intended meaning? This is the semantic problem. Third, how effectively does the received meaning affect conduct? This is the influential problem.[9] Both individual nurse professionals and the organizations they work within constantly face these communication problems.

Although we recommend that you take a look at *The Mathematical Theory of Communication* in the library, we hasten to point out that the Shannon-Weaver communication system, though illuminating, does not tell the whole story. Shannon and Weaver give the impression that communication is a one-way act starting with the sender and stopping with the receiver. They omit feedback, the response that enables the sender to adjust his or her message to the receiver. Feedback must be included in a description of the human communication process; feedback indicates the circular, ongoing nature of communication in which receivers become senders. And the concept of feedback can help solve those technical, semantic, and influential questions that Weaver raises but by no means fully answers.

Behavioral Theory

Whereas the mathematical theory Shannon developed was planned to apply to engineering or mechanical communication problems (although Weaver applied it to the wider spectrum of communication), the behavioral theory deals primarily with people, with what they perceive and think about the message, with what they think and feel on an intrapersonal, interpersonal, group, or even cultural level.

David K. Berlo's well-known SMCR (source, message, channel, receiver) model of the communication process is based on human behavior. In his 1960 text, *The Process of Communication,* Berlo carefully analyzes the ingredients[10]* necessary for communication:

SOURCE	MESSAGE	CHANNEL	RECEIVER
Communication skills	Elements	Seeing	Communication skills
Attitudes	Structure	Hearing	Attitudes
Knowledge	Content	Touching	Knowledge
Social system	Treatment	Smelling	Social system
Culture	Code	Tasting	Culture

Notice that the source and the receiver in this model appear to have the same five elements. Of course, you know that no two people are exactly alike in communication skills, attitudes, knowledge, social system, and culture. Actually, it is the differences between the source's make-up and the receiver's make-up that frequently lead to miscommunication.

Berlo's qualification that "objects which we separate may not always be separable, and they never operate independently—each affects and inter-

---

*From *The Process of Communication: An Introduction to Theory and Practice* by David Berlo. Copyright © 1960 by Holt, Rinehart and Winston, Inc. Reprinted and adapted by permission of Holt, Rinehart and Winston.

acts with the others"[11] is essential, especially as we review his useful but necessarily incomplete model of the complex communication process. In addition, his emphatic statement that "if we limit our discussion to *effective* communication, the *receiver is the most important link in the communication process*"[12] is well taken. It is somewhat surprising, however, that Berlo does not explicitly include feedback in his SMCR model. Yet he implies that feedback is an element when he refers to the interdependence of the source and the receiver during communication. And he finally treats feedback directly in a later chapter on learning.

Beyond the mathematical theory of Shannon and Weaver and the behavioral theory of Berlo, countless other versions of the communication process exist in the literature. However, the differences are slight and the similarities among them are great. Still, we should try to create the best model we can to enhance our understanding of effective communication in nursing.

A Model for the 1980s

Those who describe communication simply as the creation of a message or the making of a statement by the source are taking a message-oriented approach to communication. Those who recognize that communication requires shared experience between a sender who possesses information and a receiver who needs to know that information are taking a receiver-oriented approach. Peter F. Drucker, in *Management: Tasks, Responsibilities, Practices,* maintains that it is the recipient or perceiver who communicates, not the person who "emits" the communication.[13] What we propose for today's nurse communicators is the more realistic model shown in Figure 1.1.

Our response-oriented model includes the possibility of noise at several stages in the continuing communication process. In fact, much of this book is devoted to helping you reduce noise or barriers to effective communication. By adding feedback we have "closed the loop," for a single communication act remains incomplete without some kind of receiver response. If the sender and the receiver keep exchanging roles, the cycle of communication could be continued indefinitely. And finally, because we cannot assume that all feedback is accurate (for instance, have you ever told your instructor that you understood the day's discussion when, in fact, you didn't?), we need to test feedback, to weigh it, to find ways to determine its reliability.

As you refine your communication knowledge and skills, you should refer frequently to this response-oriented model. It can help you see the total picture, plan your communications, spot noise sources, seek and then evaluate feedback, and recall the dynamic nature of communication.

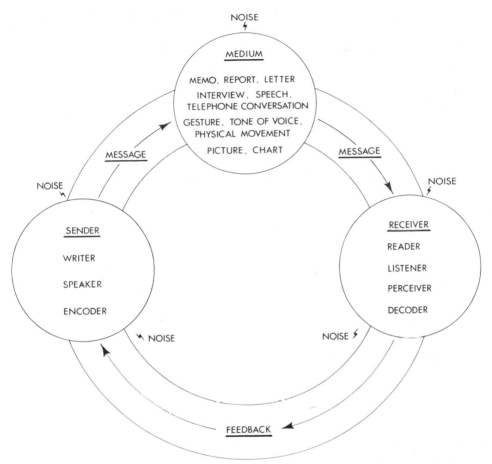

Figure 1.1. A model of the communication process, including noise and feedback.

Inappropriate Assumptions

In light of what we have said so far about the communication process and of what we shall soon say about communication barriers and facilitators, this seems like the right time to summarize the most common *inappropriate* assumptions about communication.

We are *mistaken* if we suppose that

- Communication is a simple, one-way act.
- Effective communication is easy.
- The message sent (intended) is the same as the message received (interpreted).

- People communicate only when they consciously intend to do so.
- Message receivers passively absorb messages.
- The only messages are those that are written or spoken.
- Meanings are inherent in words; thus, words mean.
- Message receivers need to be talked down to since they are not very bright.
- The sheer quantity of communication is of great importance.
- Brevity alone is the hallmark of successful communication.
- The more information, the better.
- One kind of message is appropriate for everyone.

Do you spot the flaw in each of these assumptions? Can you think of any other inappropriate assumptions about communication?

COMMUNICATION BARRIERS

The communication process is imperfect, for there are many opportunities for something to go wrong in encoding, decoding, and responding to messages in various media. That is why we built so many potential noise sources into our diagrammatic response-oriented model of the communication process. Anything that interferes with the clear and effective encoding-decoding-responding process of communication we call noise. We want you to recognize and understand the numerous barriers to communication so that you can eliminate many of them and at least cope with the remaining obstacles on somewhat more even terms than many nurses do today.

Distractions

There exist, in our professional and personal environments, many distractions that can foster communication breakdowns. Most commonly, distractions come at us through our senses. Poor lighting in a work area, an overheated classroom, a library bursting with talkative patrons, and a smoke-filled office are but a few of the noise sources we encounter daily. Next, we may be distracted by appearance, such as the poor appearance of a speaker (or an audience) or fingerprints and coffee spots on a written report. Third, the sender's or the receiver's lack of interest in the subject matter may harm the transmission of ideas. One way to secure your listeners' interest, for example, is to construct your message around the benefits they will receive if they follow your suggestions or recommendations. Lastly, we may be distracted by the countless messages that constantly compete for our attention. There are dozens of reports to be read and written, numerous nursing journals to keep up with, patients' questions to answer, and meetings to attend. We must become selective and organized or else suffer a kind of message overload. And when preparing messages, speakers or writers should realize that their messages will have to be concise, clear, and compelling enough to get through to busy listeners or readers.

Inadequate Knowledge

Another communication barrier involves inadequate knowledge on the receiver's or the sender's part. An audience of newly hired graduate nurses will probably not have sufficient background to grasp the many intricacies of a highly technical lecture on coronary care procedures by a nurse educator who has specialized in that field for years. Unless the speaker in this situation carefully analyzes the audience and adjusts the message's content and terminology accordingly, very little communication may take place. On the other hand, we sometimes find message senders who lack essential knowledge on a certain topic. If you are a graduate nurse in your first hospital assignment and one of your patients who is facing a possible radical mastectomy asks you for more information on that type of surgery's implications, you may be able to say only so much on that topic before consulting a more experienced staff member. Without the more experienced nurse's input, the patient might receive an incomplete picture.

Poor Planning and Listening

Two related and rather serious obstacles to successful communication are poor planning and careless listening.

In speaking and writing situations, it pays to plan before communicating. Organizing and presenting your ideas clearly and logically will help the reader more readily follow your written evaluation report on another team member. Are the main points made quickly and early in the report? Is there adequate development and firm support? Is the report concise without being overly abrupt? And for oral presentations, both short and long, it is helpful for listeners when you employ *purposeful* redundancy, that is, necessary repetition to overcome noise. Still appropriate today is the wise advice to, first, tell the audience in brief what you are going to tell them, then actually tell them in some detail and, finally, review what you told them.

Communication is more than writing, speaking, and reading; in fact, according to one communication expert, "about 60 percent of our time is spent listening."[14] But good listening is not easy, nor is it passive—even if the speaker offers a well-organized and apparently effective presentation. Too often, because we *think* we know what the speaker is leading up to, we race ahead to prepare our own answer or rebuttal, and in the process we may miss part of the message sent. Active listening requires effort. How often have we all blocked out sometimes important messages because we harbored preconceptions on an issue or else just would not take the time to listen carefully? Nursing practitioners who work in supervisory roles especially need to cultivate good listening skills if they are to develop their staff's potential, delegate authority, and strengthen cooperation. Of course, it is obvious that therapeutic or empathic listening enhances staff-patient communication and can play a part in promoting a client's well-being.

The positive features of planning and listening receive fuller treatment later. For now, we want to emphasize that disregarding these two crucial skills can lead to miscommunication but that it need not be this way.

Differences in Perception

From our earlier discussion of Berlo's behavioral theory of communication, you should recall that no two people are exactly alike in communication skills, attitudes, knowledge levels, and sociocultural influences. Because each of us has a mental filter and because no two mental filters are identical, it is quite common for different people to interpret a single message differently. And when they do, miscommunication results. The filter of the mind itself can be a source of noise as it accepts, alters, abstracts, and even distorts a message, situation, or event.

If two hospital staff members are present when Mr. Tompkins, a visitor, trips and falls as he steps out of the elevator, there will likely emerge two different accounts of this incident. The surgical technician who was in the elevator as Mr. Tompkins stepped out has one viewpoint; the nurse who was waiting for the elevator and who saw Mr. Tompkins's fall from that direction has another viewpoint. The differences in the reports that these two witnesses give of the same situation may be traceable to each person's unique mental filter. There is more at stake here than the fact that the surgical technician was inside the elevator and the nurse happened to be waiting outside as the doors opened and Mr. Tompkins fell. The two staff members' knowledge levels, communication skills, and the like determine what each perceives and how each will later report on the incident. For there to be effective communication about this situation, the points of view of the two witnesses need to be acknowledged, respected, and evaluated. Hopefully, Mr. Tompkins can add his version of what happened so that the causes for his fall can be understood and so that such accidents can be prevented in the future.

Another illustration of this differences-in-perception phenomenon can be seen in the aftermath of a committee meeting. Today's audit committee meeting just ended, and although everyone present supposedly *heard* the same message, already differences in interpretation of one important topic have sprung up. Fortunately, the minutes of the meeting will be available tomorrow morning to help clarify the disputed point. As accurately as possible, the secretary attempts to record proposals considered, motions passed or defeated, and areas for further discussion. But because the secretary receives and sends messages through her own mental filter, the minutes of today's meeting will be reviewed at the start of the next meeting for clarity and completeness. With feedback from the committee members, the minutes will be either accepted as submitted or accepted with corrections. Most likely, the disputed point will be clarified.

Recognizing that differences in perception play a natural part in human communication will go a long way toward making us regularly seek reliable feedback.

Emotions and Personalities

Two additional factors that can affect communication are emotions and personalities.

A nurse who is upset by a directive she has just read about new staffing policies could misinterpret or even block out parts of the morning report on her patients. The nurse's emotional reaction to one message could interfere with her reception and understanding of another message. The consequences of miscommunication during the morning report could be serious for both the nurse and her patients. If the nurse in this situation would stop to acknowledge her emotion and then try to put it in perspective *before* she participates in the morning report, the chances for better communication would be greatly improved.

Of course, sometimes emotions can play a positive role in the communication process. A clinical nurse coordinator for the medical units who starts the day in excellent spirits and who is very enthusiastic about his presentation of a series of programs to help nurses teach ostomy patients how to manage their appliances will probably succeed in getting his message across.

Akin to emotions are personalities, and more times than we care to enumerate have we seen how damaging personality conflicts can be to effective communication in a health care facility. Have you ever rejected what someone else at work has to say simply because you dislike the sender of the message? There will be little communication between one nurse and another, a nurse and a physician, or a nurse and a patient if the nurse lets the speaker's personality traits drown out that sender's message. Often the solution will be to overlook the sender's personality traits and to focus more on the message itself; often, too, it will pay off to look somewhat objectively at our own personality for the causes of communication breakdowns. It can't *always* be the other person's fault.

Frozen Evaluations

Still another contributor to miscommunication is the frozen evaluation or frozen frame of reference. Neglecting individual differences or changes with time, overemphasizing similarities, and leaping to either-or thinking characterize this communication barrier, which Haney chooses to call "differentiation failure."[15] Several examples will help you recognize and overcome this pattern of miscommunication.

When we ignore individual and important differences in the items within a group and at the same time stress only similarities, we create a stereotyped, frozen, or unfair evaluation. One hospital patient may say to his relatives that the nurse in charge of the cardiac care unit where he is now convalescing is "your *typical* head nurse." But what exactly has he communicated? What is *typical*? Certainly, head nurse 1 is not head nurse 432, yet this patient seems to be operating on the assumption that *all* head nurses are alike. A more careful statement about this head nurse's efficiency, concern, and good humor would probably be more to the point, more informative. Conversely, it is possible for a nurse to generalize unjustly about the patients in the cardiac care unit; but, of course, cardiac patient 1 is not exactly the same as cardiac patient 657 or cardiac patient 1,046. As Jane Farrell aptly points out, "When you find yourself treating patients as 'cases' rather than as people, you're showing a sure sign of Automatic Nurse Syndrome."[16] In short, we will be more in touch with reality when we remember that any person, event, or thing may be very different from others within the same general group.

As time passes and people, products, and conditions change, so also should our evaluations change. When the new head nurse of a medical floor suggests what appears to be a more equitable distribution of the work on the unit, one of the staff nurses may abruptly reply, "Well, I've been here 9 years. We never tried that plan before; I'm sure it won't work now." But perhaps the time *is right* for the new head nurse's plan to work. Perhaps the head nurse can see the larger picture, whereas the staff nurse clings to a strongly held bias that situations don't change (or shouldn't be changed). It may be that the staff nurse's static evaluation can be modified or even reversed if the head nurse explains the advantages for everybody—including the outspoken staff nurse—of at least trying out the new system. Or, for another illustration of a frozen frame of reference, consider this statement from a friend of yours: "I'll never go to Central City Hospital again . . . haven't been there since Sally was born 6 years ago . . . the floor was overcrowded and the room too hot." Most probably, hospital conditions have changed in 6 years. Central City may have added a wing and installed a climate control system. Yet your friend's statement assumes a nonchanging environment at Central City Hospital; her evaluation is based on what was true 6 years ago.

A third kind of differentiation failure involves the often hasty either-or evaluation. When we polarize, we ignore differences in degree; we allow no middle ground. Events, situations, decisions, and the like are either good or bad, black or white, happy or sad. In dealing with complex problems especially, beware of two-valued thinking, of recommending only this *or* that, of focusing on just two solutions as if there are no others. Report writers need to consider gradations between the extremes; they need to consider many possible alternatives before making a recommendation or reaching a conclusion. A nursing supervisor should take special care to avoid polarizing in an annual evaluation of a staff member. Rather than giving general praise or vague criticism, the evaluation writer should focus on the completion of specific, measurable performance goals, as well as concrete suggestions on ways the staff member can even better fulfill his or her potential.

Language

A final barrier to communication is very often language itself. There are many potential problem areas to watch out for in the system of signs and symbols that we use for communication. On the most basic level, we need to avoid common mistakes in writing and speaking. Even a relatively minor error in word choice, sentence structure, spelling, punctuation, grammar, or pronunciation will call attention to itself—and away from your real message. Throughout *Effective Communication in Nursing,* you will find helpful suggestions for overcoming errors as a source of noise so that you can achieve inconspicuousness in your writing and speaking style.

In addition, it is important to select and maintain an appropriate level of language for your specific audience. You don't want to use unnecessarily technical language in communicating with patients, for example, but neither do you want to talk down to them in a patronizing manner. Then, too, the careful use of technical/professional terminology and accepted abbreviations by nursing professionals can actually aid communication.

Bypassing, a third language-related miscommunication pattern, involves situations in which people miss each other's meanings. The more common type of bypassing occurs when the message sender and receiver assign different meanings to the same words. Another type of bypassing takes place when the sender and receiver use different words while meaning the same thing. As an illustration of bypassing, consider the following situation:

> Al Cobb in Housekeeping was having an incredibly busy Thursday. He had to speed up his routine work on 2-West—a quick mopping and buffing would have to do today—because Jim Eckles had called in sick and now Al was responsible for both 2-West and 3-North. As she was helping to pass out lunch trays, staff nurse June Logan accidentally dropped a coffeepot. Although she hastily tried to clean up the messy spill to avoid any accidents, she thought she could count on Al Cobb to finish the job after lunch. Twenty minutes later June saw Al, who was now on his way to 3-North, and said: "The floor on 2-West is a mess! Can't you do something about it?" Al returned to 2-West, redid the entire floor, never did show up on 3-North, and was called into his supervisor's office the next morning.

In fact, June wanted Al to clean up only the place where she dropped the coffeepot. She assumed that her instructions were clear, yet Al interpreted them in a wider sense and so got into trouble.

Two false assumptions about communication are at work here: (1) The message sent (intended) is the same as the message received (interpreted). (2) Meanings are inherent in words (that is, words mean). But if words *mean* anything, it is because *people* have attached meanings to them. It is more precise to say that meanings exist in the people who speak, write, hear, or read words.[17] If Al had stopped to check out his understanding of the instructions with June, or if June had been more specific and sought feedback, perhaps their miscommunication would have been avoided.

Fourth, we need to guard against the allness fallacy, that is, the false assumption that it is possible to say or to know everything about a subject. Even the most up-to-date and carefully researched journal article on alternatives to institutional care for the elderly cannot possibly cover all there is on that topic. Due to the demands of time and space, the article writer inevitably focuses on certain points while omitting less important details. We are constantly abstracting in both professional and personal communications. No incident report tells the whole story, and it is crucial that the report writer remain aware of the concepts of allness and abstracting when preparing the report. Semanticists recommend that we try adding a mental *etc.* to indicate that statements are rarely complete. In this context, moreover, it makes sense to avoid sweeping generalizations about all nurses, all patients, all doctors, all anything.

Confusing statements of inference with statements of observation is a fifth language-related trap that can lead to miscommunication. The well-known semanticist S. I. Hayakawa defines an inference as "*a statement about the unknown made on the basis of the known*. We may *infer* from the material and cut of a woman's clothes her wealth or social position; we may *infer* from the character of the ruins the origin of the fire that destroyed the building. . . . "[18] Some inferences are dependable, desirable, even necessary. When you break open a vial labeled *Furosemide* and draw up the solution for injection, you can safely assume that the vial contains this diuretic (and not something else). On the other hand, if you assume from the consistently empty meal trays that are removed from room 534 that Mr. Hanks's appetite has returned to normal, you are taking a somewhat greater risk should you consider your inference the same as verifiable fact. Perhaps Mr. Hanks's wife, who always seems to visit at mealtime, is doing most of the eating; perhaps Mr. Hanks's roommate is accepting extra portions. In order to be more certain about your appetite-return inference, you have to reassess the situation and gather more data. Why not begin to drop in on Mr. Hanks during mealtime before you accept as accurate the statement that "Mr. Hanks's appetite has returned to normal"?

ADAPTATION AS THE GATEWAY TO COMMUNICATION

Although by no means exhaustive, the preceding review of common communication barriers should help you to recognize and better cope with such potentially troublesome factors as distractions, inadequate knowledge, poor planning and listening, differences in perception, emotions and personalities, frozen evaluations, and even language itself. At this point in the discussion, we believe that you are ready to appreciate how adaptation is really the key to effective communication in nursing.

Adaptation in Nursing and in Communication

Nursing is a mutual undertaking that assists people in reaching their optimal level of wellness and in adjusting to the demands of their internal (physiological or psychological) and external (social or cultural) environments. Because nursing is a joint endeavor, one that involves both the care giver and the recipient of nursing care, it is essential that its goals be mutually understood. Yet only through the communication process can the goals of the care giver and the recipient of nursing care be understood and attained. Communication is the tool, the means, the mode of action to attain the highest level of wellness for people. We maintain that effective communication is the cornerstone for all nursing activities. Nursing is far more than the sum of its principles, interventions, or procedures. Nursing is a process depending heavily on input from the recipient of nursing care and demanding constant evaluation so that nursing activities can be adjusted or adapted to help the care giver and the recipient achieve their shared goals. In short, nursing requires adaptation, the ability to adjust to the constantly changing demands of the internal and external environments so that relevant goals are attained.

And just as nursing requires adaptation, so does effective communication. The message that the pediatric nurse sends to the toddler about not drinking or eating anything after midnight is different from the message sent to the adolescent on the same topic. In the first instance, because the toddler will most likely not understand, the message is also given to the parents and to other health care personnel, and perhaps a sign will be posted over the bed to remind others who come into contact with the toddler. In the second instance, the nurse would discuss the reason for the ban on food or liquid with the adolescent, as well as tell the other health care providers. Moreover, how the nurse treats or tailors this message will undoubtedly vary from person to person, depending on situational factors such as emotional status, intellectual ability, and readiness to learn. Obviously, then, nurses adapt their messages in light of the cues received from the patient and the environment.

The Roy Adaptation Model

Sister Callista Roy, prominent nursing theorist and educator, began to develop an adaptation model for nursing in 1964 after being challenged to construct a nursing theory framework in one of her graduate courses at the University of California, Los Angeles. Her book, *Introduction to Nursing: An Adaptation Model,* was published in 1976. Because Roy's adaptation model for nursing has much relevance to the basic principle of adaptation in communication, we will discuss her model here.

Roy sees each human being (she uses the term *man* as shorthand for both men and women) as "a biopsychosocial being in constant interaction with a changing environment."[19] This holistic viewpoint emphasizes the relatedness among diversified functions and parts within the entirety of man. Thus, man is a composite of many inseparable components in the biological, psychological, and social realms. The biological nature of man deals with the interdependence of his anatomical structure and his physiological functions. The psychological nature deals with the cognitive functions of the human being—perceiving, learning, and acting. And lastly, man's social nature refers to his behavioral patterns or interactions with other people on an interpersonal level.[20]

Roy's belief that man is an organism in constant interaction with his environment implies that adaptive measures are cyclical and exemplify change or process at every turn. The adaptation process is based on coping with various environmental changes. The organism that cannot adapt to environmental stressors will not survive very long. But any environmental changes will require responses that, hopefully, are adaptive. In other words, adaptive responses are efficient, effective, and helpful in propelling man forward to attain new heights physically, psychologically, and socially. Man's potential to achieve his fullest psychological and spiritual development is almost unlimited.[21]

Figure 1.2 illustrates one of the assumptions underlying the adaptation process, for if man successfully interacts with his changing environment, the messages that return to him from the environment—the feedback—help him adapt or modify his behavior to attain his goals. Since man constantly interacts with his environment, he adapts to forces that shape, mold, and influence him. Nursing communication, therefore, becomes an integral part of the adaptation process. Adaptive nursing communication embraces (1) the sum of those messages that the client or the nurse initiates or receives and (2) how the individual adapts his messages as he interacts with a fluctuating environment.

Another important assumption underlying Roy's model is that man

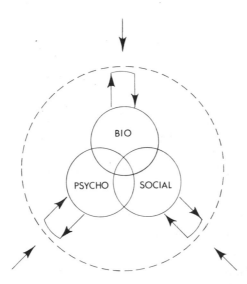

Figure 1.2. Man as a biopsychosocial being in constant interaction with a changing environment.

uses both innate and acquired mechanisms that are biological, psychological, and social to cope with the changing world. Innate mechanisms, or those belonging to the individual at birth, include unconscious biological responses. The normal physiological response to a superficial cut, for instance, is vasoconstriction followed by platelet formation. Acquired mechanisms or learned responses include psychological defense mechanisms such as denial, repression, or projection. Discovering a lump in one's breast is a stressful situation that provokes such an intolerably high level of anxiety that the person may well block it out by denial. Social mechanisms that enable man to exist comfortably in the environment include all forms of communication and those culturally defined patterns that formalize our interpersonal interactions.

Roy's Model and Adaptive Communication

What, then, are the implications of Roy's adaptation model for nursing communication? Because we accept the premise that man is a biopsychosocial being, we maintain that he or she communicates in all three modes—biological, psychological, and social. Although biological communication seems the most basic, it cannot be overlooked as an integral component of nonverbal communication. Biological responses communicate; they send forth messages about the body's physiological state. The physiological signs of shock such as pallor, cyanosis, and clammy extremities communicate far more to the prudent nurse in many circumstances than do more formal communication channels. Social indicators arise from man's social component; they include socially accepted and culturally determined modes of formal communication such as reading, writing, listening, and speaking, as well as gestures, signs, and extralinguistic phenomena like pitch, tone, and affect. As for the psychological mode, we can communicate moods and feelings both verbally and nonverbally.

The principle of adaptation as applied to nursing communication may be summarized as follows: The communicator adapts his or her message to best fit the needs and demands of a constantly changing environment. Environmental factors to consider in encoding might include such variables as

- Group size
- Cultural or ethnic background
- Educational or maturational level
- Psychosocial factors
- Physiological problems
- Amount of time available

To clarify further what adapting a message to a receiver (usually a listener or a reader) in a nursing context means, let's return to the message about the ban on food or liquid that the pediatric nurse must send to both the toddler and the adolescent.

The pediatric nurse wants to transmit the message so that both children understand. But as we pointed out earlier, this nurse will carefully adapt or modify the message according to environmental cues. For 4-year-old Alicia, the oldest child of Chicano migrant workers, the nurse weighs the child's maturational level, the parents' and their daughter's ability to understand and speak English, the sensory deficit (impaired hearing) of Alicia's father, the physiological problem (generalized lower abdominal pain) that Alicia is experiencing, and the size of the group (Alicia, both parents, an aunt and uncle) when preparing this deceptively "simple" message. Clearly, this is a more complex communication problem than sending similar message content to a high school freshman who has no sensory impairments, whose physiological integrity remains intact, and who is from the same sociocultural background as the nurse.

Yet another problem in adaptive nursing communication persists on 4-East at Fieldcrest Memorial Hospital for nurses who have to communicate various kinds of information each workday. Foremost is sending and receiving information during the change-of-shift report. Information that is vital for the continuity of patient care must be exchanged. But just how is it to be sent most effectively? What environmental factors should be taken into account to ensure that it has a high probability of being understood by nurses on the next shift? Items to consider include the limits of time, the levels of employees hearing the report, the place where the report is made, and the kind and amount of information that should be conveyed. A nurse who reports to an all-professional staff plans and sends one type of message. But if a nurse is speaking (or writing) to a mixed group of professional and ancillary personnel, the message's wording, structure, and content will change. In each case, the nurse modifies or adapts a particular message for a particular audience.

COMMUNICATION FACILITATORS

A message that is carefully adapted to the receiver's knowledge, interests, and experience tends to be effective because it fits the receiver, who feels as if the message was created especially for him. Planned presentation, you-viewpoint, and appropriate language are the three preeminent communication facilitators that derive from the basic principle of adaptation. Before moving on to the many nursing communication challenges and situations treated in succeeding chapters, we want to introduce, albeit briefly, these three facilitators, which play such a significant role in achieving better written communication (an area in which nursing professionals often need the most help) and nonwritten communication.

Planned Presentation

Planning before communicating saves time in the long run for busy message senders and receivers because it simultaneously increases the likelihood of an effective communication having a minimum amount of noise. When you have a speech or talk to prepare and present, the place to start is with the following preparatory steps. Many people have heard of these or similar planning steps, but too few communicators consistently employ them. If you are asked to speak on the rehabilitation needs of the cardiac patient, (1) determine your message's purpose and (2) identify your audience. Then, in light of the first two steps, you can proceed to (3) decide which main points to include and (4) gather the necessary details and facts to support your main points. The next step is to (5) order your thoughts for best reception by the audience. Usually, the direct structure (big idea, explanation, summary) works well when you want to give primary attention to the facts. But sometimes, especially in bad-news and persuasive situations, you may use the indirect approach in which the big idea is delayed until you first establish a pleasant emotional tone. Only now should you (6) write the draft and (7) polish and practice your talk until you are ready to communicate with your audience.

You-Viewpoint

You-viewpoint or you-attitude means seeing and presenting a nursing communication situation from the receiver's point of view. It is an attitude or state of mind that leads you to focus on the message receiver's needs, interests, and way of looking at the world. One characteristic of the you-viewpoint is that it uses more second person pronouns (*you, your*) than first person pronouns (*I, we, our,* etc.). Another characteristic is that it emphasizes the positive aspects of any situation.

In reviewing the viewpoint examples on page 29, you should notice how the version on the right focuses on the receiver's viewpoint and also highlights a benefit for the receiver.

Appropriate Language

The third communication facilitator that follows logically from the principle of adaptation is appropriate language. At this stage, we can best

Sender Viewpoint	*Receiver Viewpoint*
I have 6 years' experience in psychiatric nursing.	My 6 years' experience in psychiatric nursing would enable me to make an effective contribution to your new psychiatric unit.
I have approved your request for 2 weeks' vacation starting July 15.	Yes, you may begin your 2 weeks' vacation on July 15.
You neglected to fill in your selections for breakfast, lunch, and dinner tomorrow.	To enjoy tomorrow's menu as much as possible, you should fill in your breakfast, lunch, and dinner selections.
I want to send my congratulations to you for completing 20 years of continuous service.	Congratulations on your 20 years of continuous service.
Our Peoria Hospital Development Fund is trying to raise money for improvements in the snack bar and gift shop. We can achieve our goal if you will help us. We need to have all pledges of support in our office by October 1 if we are to have time to process them by October 15.	You can help meet the goal of improving the snack bar and gift shop by making your pledge to the Peoria Hospital Development Fund by October 1.
Our policy prohibits us from permitting more than two visitors per patient at any one time.	So that your recovery may be speedy, we ask that you have just one or two visitors at a time.

introduce you to this complex communication pathway through selected examples.

On one level, appropriate language refers to careful and economical word choice that combats what Edith P. Lewis, in a *Nursing Outlook* editorial, calls the "syndrome of pretentious prose."[22] On page 30 is an incomplete list of wordy, trite, or stereotyped expressions to be avoided. Can you add some of your own?

On another level, appropriate language recognizes the needs of and the differences between technical and general audiences. Although "NPO for UGI" would be an acceptable entry on a patient's chart, a nurse could profitably translate that phrase as follows, when talking to the patient, Mr. Bliss, who is not a health professional: "Mr. Bliss, you won't be able to have anything to eat or drink until you come back from your stomach x-ray. But as soon as you return, I'll order your breakfast."

Instead of This	*Say This*
seven in number	seven
arrived at the conclusion	concluded
conceptualize	think of
initiate	begin
at this point in time	now
a multiplicity of reasons	many reasons
reason is because	because
in regard to	about
underlying basis	basis
surrounding environment	environment
scoliosis of the spine	scoliosis
onset of menarche	menarche
in the final analysis	finally
along the lines of	like
male nurse	nurse
chairman	chairperson
lady doctor	doctor
manmade	artificial

And a third way of looking at appropriate language concerns the elements of specificity and completeness. Notice that the abrupt entry on a chart, "Ambulated in hall," is not as complete, detailed, or accurate as the revised entry: "Ambulated length of north hall with assistance of nurse. Some dyspnea noted on return to room, but Ms. Johns voluntarily used pursed-lip breathing to compensate. Respirations rose from 20 to 26 on return to room." In another pairing, the more accurate statement, "Incision clean and dry. Edges approximated. No redness or discoloration. Granulation tissue present," clearly improves on the shorter, hopelessly relative statement, "Incision healing." Conciseness—not to be confused with excessive brevity—means transmitting your message in the fewest possible words while still being specific and including all relevant details.

SUMMARY

In laying the theoretical foundation for the study of effective communication in nursing, we discover that communication is the essence of nursing, *the* tool with which to accomplish patient care goals. The nursing communication situations that arise in just a single workday are many and varied; yet the potential for miscommunication—whether in written, oral, or nonverbal messages—is always present.

Communication is important in meeting organizational goals, in satisfying professional responsibilities, and in fulfilling personal roles.

To inquire, to inform, to persuade, and to entertain are the four purposes of communication.

Effective communication can be measured in terms of whether or not the sender's message has had the intended impact on its receiver. Real communication occurs when the receiver provides some response to the sender through feedback.

Theories and models prove useful in studying the complex process of communication. The mathematical theory and the behavioral theory can start you on the way to becoming a better nurse communicator. Our response-oriented communication model for the 1980s includes noise and feedback and should be referred to frequently as you refine your communication knowledge and skills.

The communication barriers to recognize, understand, and eliminate or at least cope with fall into seven basic categories: (1) distractions, (2) inadequate knowledge, (3) poor planning and listening, (4) differences in perception, (5) emotions and personalities, (6) frozen evaluations, and (7) language itself.

Adaptation is the key to effective communication in nursing. Roy's adaptation model can be applied to nursing communication. In this scheme, the communicator adapts his or her message to best fit the needs and demands of a constantly changing environment. In short, the nurse purposefully modifies or adapts a particular message for a particular audience.

Three preeminent communication facilitators that derive from the basic principle of adaptation are (1) planned presentation, (2) you-viewpoint, and (3) appropriate language. These facilitators play a significant role in achieving better written and nonwritten communications, as you will see from the many nursing communication challenges and situations treated in succeeding chapters.

EXERCISES

1. Discuss the meaning of the following communication terms or concepts. In order to clarify your definitions, cite an original example from your own experience for each item listed.
   - Communication model
   - Feedback
   - Communication barrier

- Mental filter
- Frozen evaluation
- Bypassing
- Adaptive communication
- You-viewpoint
- Planned presentation
- Appropriate language

2. Compare and contrast the mathematical theory of communication with the behavioral theory of communication. Does either tell the whole story?

3. Construct your own definition of communication. Write it down and save it until the last week of this course. Then review it to see whether or not you need to change it.

4. Give several examples of how emotions and personalities can affect communication.

5. Which of the following are statements of inference? Which are statements of observation or verifiable fact? Defend your responses.

   a. Air Cushion shoes are no good.

   b. Bill Lowry, the new nurse anesthetist, is a "loser."

   c. The new increases bring starting salaries for staff nurses to $1,196 a month.

   d. The new increases in monthly salaries for beginning staff nurses are still too small.

6. How much of your time do you spend communicating? Tomorrow, keep a diary of your communication activities from the time you wake up until the time you retire. What kinds of communication activities did you engage in? What were some of the purposes of these communications? Which communications were successful? Which were unsuccessful? Prepare a short oral report of your findings to share with the class.

7. Try to picture one person with whom you have some trouble communicating effectively. First, identify that person (perhaps a relative or friend). Next, list the barriers that make communication between the two of you at times difficult. Finally, propose some solutions for overcoming noise.

8. Bring to class sufficient photocopies of a cartoon that contains numerous details. Allow your classmates 1 minute to observe the cartoon and then ask them to write a concise description of what they saw. As three or four volunteers read their descriptions, you and the class should spot differences in perception. Does any single description cover all the details in the cartoon?

9. Select from a recent nursing publication an article dealing with communication problems and practices and write a 500-word review of it.

10. Spend a half-hour in a health care facility observing the communication activities of the people (especially nursing personnel) present. These activities could include writing, speaking, reading, and listening. In addition, do you observe any nonverbal communication elements such as gestures, tone of voice, or physical movements? Take notes and then write a 300-word report describing the communication (or miscommunication) you observed.

11. Prepare six quiz questions for this chapter. Test these questions on the members of your small discussion group. Does miscommunication occur? Can you correct the question(s) to overcome this?

REFERENCES

1. William V. Haney, *Communication and Interpersonal Relations,* 4th ed. (Homewood, IL: Irwin, 1979), p. 3.
2. Haney, p. 3.
3. John Fielden, "What Do You Mean I Can't Write?" *Harvard Business Review,* 42 (May–June 1964), 144–145.
4. Eleanor C. Hein, *Communication in Nursing Practice* (Boston: Little, Brown, 1973), p. 22.
5. David S. Fuller and Gustavo M. Quesada, "Communication in Medical Therapeutics," *The Journal of Communication,* 23 (December 1973), 361.
6. David K. Berlo, *The Process of Communication: An Introduction to Theory and Practice* (New York: Holt, Rinehart and Winston, 1960), p. 24.
7. Francis W. Weeks and Daphne A. Jameson, *Principles of Business Communication,* 2d ed. (Champaign, IL: Stipes, 1979), p. 20.
8. Claude E. Shannon and Warren Weaver, *The Mathematical Theory of Communication* (Urbana, IL: University of Illinois Press, 1949), p. 98.
9. Shannon and Weaver, p. 96.
10. Berlo, p. 72.
11. Berlo, p. 26.
12. Berlo, p. 52.
13. Peter F. Drucker, *Management: Tasks, Responsibilities, Practices* (New York: Harper & Row, 1973), p. 483.
14. Norman B. Sigband, *Communication for Management and Business,* 2d ed. (Glenview, IL: Scott, Foresman, 1976), p. 14.
15. Haney, p. 387.
16. Jane Farrell, "The Human Side of Assessment," *Nursing80,* 10 (April 1980), 74.

17. Haney, p. 586. See also the essay "How Words Change Our Lives" by S. I. Hayakawa in *Symbol, Status, and Personality* (New York: Harcourt, Brace and World, 1958), pp. 3–17, for a helpful introduction to general semantics.
18. S. I. Hayakawa, *Language in Thought and Action,* 4th ed. (New York: Harcourt Brace Jovanovich, 1978), p. 35.
19. Sister Callista Roy, *Introduction to Nursing: An Adaptation Model* (Englewood Cliffs, NJ: Prentice-Hall, 1976), p. 11.
20. Roy, pp. 3–19.
21. Abraham H. Maslow in *Motivation and Personality,* 2d ed. (New York: Harper & Row, 1970), pp. 35–58, outlines a hierarchy of human needs with five levels: (1) physiological needs, (2) safety and security needs, (3) social needs, (4) ego needs, and (5) self-actualization needs. Roy cites Maslow's theory and builds on it.
22. Edith P. Lewis, "Pretentious Prose," *Nursing Outlook,* 22 (July 1974), 431.

FURTHER READING

Barnlund, Dean C. "Toward a Meaning-centered Philosophy of Communication." *The Journal of Communication,* 12 (1962), 197–211.

Bowen-Jones, Jane. "Therapeutic Communication: The Nurse's Counselling Role." *The Australian Nurses' Journal,* 8 (June 1979), 54–56.

Brunner, Nancy A. "Communications in Nursing Service Administration." *Journal of Nursing Administration,* 7 (October 1977), 29–32.

Campbell, James H., and Hal W. Hepler, eds. *Dimensions in Communication,* 2d ed. Belmont, CA: Wadsworth, 1971.

Dance, Frank E. X. "The 'Concept' of Communication." *The Journal of Communication,* 20 (June 1970), 201–210.

Huseman, Richard C., Cal M. Logue, and Dwight L. Freshley, eds. *Readings in Interpersonal and Organizational Communication,* 2d ed. Boston: Holbrook, 1973.

Le Roux, Rose S. "Communication and Influence in Nursing." *Nursing Administration Quarterly,* 2 (Spring 1978), 51–57.

Lynaugh, Joan E., and Barbara Bates. "The Two Languages of Nursing and Medicine." *American Journal of Nursing,* 73 (January 1973), 66–69.

Mortensen, C. David. *Basic Readings in Communication Theory.* New York: Harper & Row, 1973.

Rosendahl, Pearl L. "The Verbal Side of Effective Communication." *Journal of Nursing Administration,* 4 (September–October 1974), 41–44.

Skipper, James K., Jr., Hans O. Mauksch, and Daisy Tagliacozzo. "Some Barriers to Communication Between Patients and Hospital Functionaries." *Nursing Forum,* 2 (1963), 14–23.

Wang, Rosemary Y., and Joellen Watson Hawkins. "Interpersonal Feedback for Nursing Supervisors." *Supervisor Nurse,* 11 (January 1980), 26–28.

CHAPTER II

Client-Centered Documentation Within the Nursing Process

Objectives

After studying this chapter, you will be able to

1. Explain the relationship between the process of documentation and the nursing process.
2. Differentiate between nursing histories and nursing assessments.
3. Write meaningful nursing assessments and nursing diagnoses.
4. State the importance of writing client-centered care plans.
5. List the components of care plans.
6. Write effective client-centered care plans, including short-term goals, long-term goals, and nursing orders.
7. Critique selected teaching plan formats.
8. Write a teaching plan that demonstrates the relationship between learner objectives and teaching activities.
9. Write measurable learner-oriented performance objectives.
10. Differentiate between the source-oriented and the problem-oriented documentation systems.
11. State general guidelines for effective documentation.
12. Write meaningful narrative progress notes.
13. Write progress notes using the problem-oriented format.
14. Write three types of discharge summaries.

From nursing histories to discharge summaries, there is a wide variety of types of documentation that nurses in health care agencies must prepare about clients. Because we believe that the basis of effective client-centered documentation is the nursing process, we provide a brief overview of that process before discussing in detail the principles and guidelines for writing nursing histories and assessments, nursing diagnoses, care plans, teaching plans, meaningful objectives, documentation systems, and discharge summaries.

THE NURSING PROCESS

The nursing process forms the framework for all nursing activities, including the written results of those activities; it is the application of the scientific method of problem solving to client care. Because the term *process* denotes a series of events that are interrelated, interdependent, and cyclical, none of the phases of the nursing process can stand alone and have full meaning. Assessment, planning, implementation, and evaluation are the four steps of the nursing process.

Assessment

Assessment, the first phase of the nursing process, can be considered the catalyst or initiator of the problem-solving cycle. In this phase, information is gathered about the client's biopsychosocial status and his or her activities of daily living. Assessment provides the rationale for identifying the client's problems and serves as a basis for formulating a nursing diagnosis. Important sources of information that contribute to the assessment stage include nursing histories and assessments, medical histories and physical examinations, formal and informal interviews with the client's family, the client's present and past medical records, and planned or casual observations of the client's reaction to stressors.

Since the potential scope of data in the assessment phase is substantial, the nurse must analyze and interpret the data to make nursing diagnoses. Nursing diagnoses are concise statements, based on a synthesis of the data collected in the assessment phase, that describe a client's actual or potential health problems and the factors that could be related to the origin of the problems. Nursing diagnoses, then, describe problems that professional nurses, by virtue of their educational preparation, are capable of treating.

We should remember, moreover, that although assessment always begins the nursing process and always leads to a nursing diagnosis, continuous assessment (or reassessment—the additional gathering and analysis of data) can occur during the planning, implementation, and evaluation stages. New information obtained through reassessment may even lead to a change in the original nursing diagnosis. In sum, the assessment phase both initiates the nursing process and serves as a source of continuing data for the problem-solving system.

Planning

Planning, the organizational phase of the nursing process, involves setting goals and objectives, judging priorities, and designing methods to resolve problems. The written care plan, the direct and concrete result of the planning stage, provides consistency and continuity of care. Planning must be based on the assessment phase and the nursing diagnosis, or else the unique needs of the client may not be met. One crucial aspect of the planning phase is goal setting, that is, establishing a specific target date by which each long- or short-term goal can realistically be expected to be attained. Whenever possible, the client should be an active participant in the planning step so that compliance in attaining the goals of the treatment regimen is enhanced.

Implementation

During the implementation phase, the nurse intervenes by initiating or completing nursing actions that meet the goals and objectives of resolving the client's problems. Usually, implementation means the actual giving or delivery of nursing care. It consists of nursing therapy (for example, the therapeutic use of touch), nursing treatments, various therapeutic communication techniques, the physician's medical regimen, and health education programs. During this phase, too, the nurse is frequently engaged in documenting on the client's record the results of interventions. Understanding two commonly used documentation systems (discussed later in this chapter) can help the nurse effectively record interventions.

Evaluation

The fourth phase is evaluation, the judgment phase of the nursing process, in which the nurse determines to what extent nursing intervention has been successful in preventing or resolving the client's problems and in meeting long- or short-term goals. Questions the nurse should ask during the evaluation phase include the following:

- Was the care I gave effective? Why? Why not?
- Were the goals and objectives clearly stated?
- Were the goals and objectives met? Have I seen changes in the client's behavior?
- Was I able to predict the outcome of my nursing actions?

Evaluation is the most dynamic of the four phases, for it not only applies to each of the four steps separately but also applies to the entire nursing process itself. How well was each step, including the evaluation phase, performed? How successful was the entire nursing process? And so if one care plan is not successful, another plan may be developed; or perhaps the original plan may become successful after undergoing various modifications.

The basis of appropriate evaluation lies in the planning stage. If short-term goals (objectives) are clearly stated in specific behavioral terms, it is relatively easy to determine where the client stands in relation to the achievement of the goal. According to Dolores E. Little and Doris L. Carnevali, evaluation consists of three sequential steps to determine to what extent the client has moved toward a mutually defined goal:

1. Selecting standards related to specific client behaviors
2. Collecting data *after* goals have been set and interventions have occurred, as evidence of whether goals and objectives were met
3. Comparing the collected evidence to the criteria and baseline data, if they are available, and making judgments about the nature of the client's behavioral changes[1]

The nurse's role in documenting the evaluation phase requires recording the evaluation of care in the evaluation column of the care plan, reformulating short-term goals if the first ones were not successful or could not be attained, and documenting the client's response to nursing and medical care, via the discharge summary on the clinical record. As part of the evaluation phase, the nurse may also take part in the nursing audit, which authorities such as Maria C. Phaneuf describe as the systematic written appraisal of the quality of nursing care as indicated by the clinical records of discharged clients.[2]

NURSING ASSESSMENTS

To deal effectively with clients when they enter the health care system, the nurse first has to know exactly what the clients' needs or problems are. Therefore, the careful recording of data collected during the nursing interview becomes extremely important to the problem-solving process, for it becomes the baseline assessment from which to identify problems, formulate a nursing diagnosis, and plan the client's care.

Nursing Histories Versus Nursing Assessments

Nurses use nursing histories and nursing assessments as methodological tools to gather baseline data about their clients. The difference between histories and assessments is mainly one of scope. Typically, the nursing history focuses on subjective data, such as the client's health history, sociocultural status, lifestyle, activities of daily living, and perceptions of self and his or her health status. But when the data collection process *also* encompasses the nurse's observation of selected physical findings, nonverbal communication patterns, and extralinguistic phenomena (such as pitch, tone of voice, crying), as well as the use of touch in palpation and percussion, then the term *nursing assessment* better fits the activity. Since it incorporates the gathering of both subjective (history-taking) data and objective (observational) data, we prefer Little and Carnevali's definition of the nursing assessment as "a focused, time-limited interaction between a nurse and a client with the purpose of collecting subjective and objective data needed to effectively plan nursing's participation in this client's health care management."[3]

The actual content of the nursing assessment varies from agency to agency, depending on agency needs and client population. Nevertheless, Ann Marriner suggests four general categories: (1) activities of daily living, including hygiene routines, elimination habits, dietary patterns, exercise, and sleep habits; (2) physical status, including level of consciousness, sensory status, and modes of adaptation to sensory deficits; (3) psychological status; and (4) social-cultural-economic history, including the client's understanding of his or her present health, reaction to previous health care, and expectations of the present health care system.[4]

Furthermore, Little and Carnevali identify two key areas that they consider basic to all nursing assessments written in any type of health care facility: (1) the coping challenges to effective living and optimal health and (2) the available resources and abilities that enable the client to deal with the coping challenges.[5] They then recommend collecting data on the client's perception of these coping challenges (current health status, goals, needed and usable services, etc.), the client's functional abilities (breathing and circulation, elimination, emotional factors, mobility, sexuality, etc.), and external resources and support systems (housing, transportation, schools, family networks, friends, etc.). Yet perhaps even more useful to review at this point in the discussion are the major headings for nursing assessments proposed by Marjory Gordon at the 1979 New England Regional Conference on Nursing Diagnosis and cited by Derry A. Moritz in a recent *Oncology Nursing Forum* article:

1. Nutritional/metabolic patterns
2. Sleep/rest patterns
3. Activity/exercise patterns
4. Elimination patterns
5. Immunological competence
6. Sexual/reproductive patterns
7. Role/relationship
8. Cognitive/perceptual patterns
9. Communication patterns
10. Coping pattern/stress tolerance
11. Self-perception
12. Illness/health–belief systems
13. Life patterns/lifestyle[6]

Although the nurse customarily uses the agency's form to document nursing histories and assessments, we hasten to emphasize that the essence of the nursing assessment is *not* the form. On the contrary, the nursing assessment represents the initial phase of the nursing process and serves as a tool to help the nurse collect data in an efficient manner in order to reach a nursing diagnosis and to plan client-centered care. Nevertheless, an appropriately structured format helps nurses to interview clients and write meaningful assessments without overlooking key content areas. When nurses work with a particular client population (for example, adult oncology patients), a specially designed assessment form or "tool"[7] can sensibly limit the quantity of information collected because it focuses on the most likely problem areas.

Today, formats for nursing assessments range from the structured checklist (Exhibit 2.1) to the nearly blank sheet of paper with very few headings. Currently, semistructured formats (Exhibit 2.2) are popular since they help writers decide what kind of information to include yet are sufficiently flexible so that nurses with varying levels of education and experience can use them.[8] The more "open" assessment format with few headings or cues receives support from Little and Carnevali, for two reasons. First, such a tool recognizes that not all clients are hospitalized and so has a wider application for nurses who work in home health agencies, outpatient clinics, and rehabilitation centers. Second, because more nurses are now familiar with nursing assessment, either through basic education or continuing education courses, the cues that the more structured checklist provides are not necessary—in fact, they may inhibit nurses' creativity.[9]

Guidelines for Writing Nursing Assessments

Whatever type of nursing assessment tool you use, you should be familiar enough with it so that it serves as a *guide* to the interviewing and data collection process. Methodological tools, like other tools, should work *for* you—you should not be so strictly bound to them that you are a captive of the tool designed to help you.

The decision about *when* to record the assessment is often influenced by the amount of time available and by the nurse's ability and desire to combine interviewing and writing. Through role-playing situations, Little and Carnevali found that although some nurses believe clients become uncomfortable when the nurse records or takes notes during the nursing assessment interview, it is actually the nurse who feels uncomfortable. They suggest telling the client at the beginning of the interview that you will be taking notes to help you remember pertinent dates, medi-

BARBERTON CITIZENS HOSPITAL
NURSING ADMISSION ASSESSMENT & HISTORY

Arrival: Date_____ Time_____ to room_____

From _____

Walking_____ Wheel Chair_____ Stretcher_____

First BCH Admission Yes_____ No_____

PATIENT'S/FAMILY REASON FOR THIS ADMISSION:

Family Physician _____

_____

_____

PATIENT'S PAST MEDICAL HISTORY - HAS PATIENT EVER HAD ANY OF FOLLOWING DISEASES?

LUNG DISEASE
____ Asthma
____ Bronchitis
____ Tuberculosis
____ Emphysema
____ Lung Cancer
____ Smokers cough

HEART DISEASE
____ Heart attack
____ Angina (Pain)
____ Palpitations
____ High BP
____ Heart Failure
____ Shortness of breath
____ Rheumatic fever
____ Heart murmur
____ Severe ankle swelling
____ Leakage of heart valve
____ Other _____

PREVIOUS SURGERIES (Date)
____ Tonsil _____
____ Appendix _____
____ Hernia _____
____ Gallbladder _____
____ Stomach _____
____ Bowel _____
____ Other _____
____ Most recent surgery _____

KIDNEY DISEASE
____ Nephritis or nephrosis
____ Bloody urine
____ Kidney stone
____ Prostate trouble
____ Difficulty in urinating
____ No bladder control
____ Other _____

CENTRAL NERVOUS SYSTEM DISEASE
____ Stroke
____ Polio
____ Paralysis
____ Meningitis
____ Migraine headache
____ Convulsions
____ Multiple sclerosis
____ Mental illness
____ Other _____

____ D&C _____
____ Breast _____
____ Hysterectomy _____
____ Back surgery _____
____ Kidneystone _____
____ Lung surgery _____

LIVER DISEASE
____ Jaundice
____ Cirrhosis
____ Hepatitis

GI TRACT DISEASE
____ Ulcer
____ Spastic colon
____ Colitis
____ Diverticulitis
____ Bowel obstruction
____ Rectal bleeding
____ Other _____

MISCELLANEOUS
____ Diabetes
____ Thyroid disease
____ Arthritis
____ Anemia
____ Other _____

PREVIOUS ANESTHETICS
____ Pentothal
____ Gas
____ Spinal
____ Nerve block
____ Other _____
____ Any problems _____

ARE YOU ALLERGIC TO ANY MEDICATIONS?
Yes_____ No_____

PATIENT'S MEDICAL HISTORY-AT PRESENT TIME
____ Any recent acute illness such as:
____ Chest cold
____ Sinus infection
____ Weight loss
____ Elevated temperature

Are you presently being treated for:
____ Chronic lung condition
____ Heart condition
____ Liver disease
____ Kidney disease

_____

_____

How much do you smoke per day?

_____

ARE YOU PRESENTLY TAKING MEDICATIONS (OR HAVE YOU TAKEN WITHIN PAST 6 MONTHS)

____ Digitalis preparation   ____ Eye Meds
____ Diuretics
____ High blood pressure pills
____ Nitroglycerin
____ Insulin or oral diabetic med.
____ Tranquilizers
____ Cortisone
____ Iron
____ Weight control pills
____ Blood thinners
____ Vasodilators
____ Other _____

How much do you drink per day?

_____

Do you have any loose teeth, partials,
bridges, or caps?

_____

_____

2755 (8-77)

Exhibit 2.1. Structured checklist for a nursing assessment (front).

43

NURSING ASSESSMENT

WEIGHT_____ HEIGHT_____
Wt./ht. deferred because

PULSE rate radial_____ apical_____ other_____

    rhythm: regular_____ irregular_____ quality_____

    If patient has a pacemaker, indicate type: perm._____ temp._____

BLOOD PRESSURE right arm_____ left arm_____

ALLERGIES: Other than medications

TEMPERATURE oral_____ rectal_____ axillary_____

RESPIRATION rate_____per min.

    character:

    coughing_____ producing sputum_____

    receiving oxygen per mask_____ cannula_____

    has chest tubes_____ has tracheostomy_____

    Ventilation aide(s) in use:

N U T R I T I O N & E L I M I N A T I O N

wearing dentures_____ edentulous_____
mouth condition:

home diet _____

food intolerances _____

time of last oral intake_____ solids_____ liquids_____

nauseated_____ vomiting_____ anorexic_____

tube feeding amount: nasogastric_____ gastrostomy_____

---

frequency of stool_____liquid_____soft_____hard_____diarrhea_____

constipated: uses laxative_____type:_____enema_____

incontinence_____frequency_____retention_____burning with urination_____

date of last catheter change _____

Ostomy home care routine:
Bowel   Bladder

S K I N

               Location/Size

Rash _____ | Localized swelling _____

Abrasion _____ | Ulcer _____

Discoloration_____ | Other _____

Edema _____

Comments about: duration, pain, itching, home treatment, etc.

S E N S E S

wearing: glasses_____ contacts_____ eye prosthesis_____

wearing a hearing aid_____

Comments about sight or hearing conditions, patterns of speech & communication, etc.

B E H A V I O R

alert & oriented_____ Combative_____

not oriented to: time_____ person_____ place_____

lethargic_____ confused_____ unresponsive_____

Comments about patient's attitude, mood, behavioral changes, etc.

ACTIVITIES OF DAILY LIVING: independent_____

    Needs assistance with eating_____ bathing_____

    dressing/grooming_____ walking_____

    Aides used for mobility:

    Sleep/rest patterns or difficulties:

    Patient lives alone_____ with family_____

    in nursing home_____ other_____

---

occupation, interests, etc.

Medicine brought to hospital was:

sent home_____ given to pharmacy_____ kept in room_____

PAIN:

List problems from information obtained on appropriate form.

                                             a.m.

Dr._____ notified at_____ p.m. of patient's admission.

Nurse's Signature

Exhibit 2.1. Structured checklist for a nursing assessment (back).

Exhibit 2.2. Semistructured format for a nursing assessment (front).

NURSING HISTORY AND	NAME
ADMISSION ASSESSMENT	AGE
	ADDRESS
	PHYSICIAN
	IDENTIFICATION NUMBER

CHIEF COMPLAINT/REASON FOR CONTACT (use client's own words)

HISTORY OF CURRENT ILLNESS

PAST MEDICAL PROBLEMS/SURGERIES (include reaction to illness)

FAMILY HISTORY (include hereditary or chronic diseases)

CURRENT MEDICATIONS (include ASA, oral contraceptives, laxatives, other OTC preparations)

ALLERGIES (food, drugs, environmental agents)

PATIENT PROFILE

    MARITAL STATUS   S   M   D   W   Sep

    CLOSE FAMILY MEMBERS/SIGNIFICANT OTHERS

    OCCUPATION

    RELIGION

    HOME (description, location, with whom client lives)

Exhibit 2.2. Semistructured format for a nursing assessment (back).

HOBBIES/INTERESTS

EDUCATION

HABITS (drugs, alcohol, coffee, tobacco)

EFFECT OF ILLNESS ON LIFESTYLE/FAMILY

REVIEW OF SYSTEMS AND HEALTH STATUS (use *S* to indicate information from client/family and *O* to indicate your own observations)

1. Vision

2. Hearing

3. Speech

4. ADL (include adaptive or coping mechanisms)

5. Skin/hygiene

6. Sleep/rest

7. Cardiovascular

8. Respiratory

9. Gastrointestinal (nutrition, bowel elimination)

10. Genitourinary (bladder and reproductive functioning)

11. Musculoskeletal

12. Psychosocial

HEALTH MAINTENANCE RECORD

DATE AND RESULTS OF:

PAP TEST _____ CHEST X-RAY _____

EKG _____ DENTAL EXAM _____

EYE EXAM _____ BREAST SELF-EXAM _____

PHYSICAL EXAM _____

_____ R.N.

cations, and the like. Through role playing and actual clinical experience, these same authors also discovered that the nurse and the client both felt more comfortable during the recording process when they were seated in the same direction. This way, the client could see what the nurse was writing. A measure that may help when the seating arrangements do not permit the client to see what the nurse is writing is to comment aloud on what is being recorded. Little and Carnevali observed that permitting the client to know what was being recorded "increased the sense of working together in the management of health problems and reduced the sense of the secrecy of health records."[10]

Whether you use a checklist, an open format with few headings, or a semistructured format to record a nursing assessment, there are 10 basic guidelines that apply to the process.

Guideline 1

Avoid using *client* or *patient* in the assessment since the record refers to the client. When necessary for clarity, use the person's initials—"Mr. J.," "Ms. K. C.," "Mrs. P.," or simply "J. D."

Guideline 2

Record the dates, places, and unusual circumstances of all previous surgeries, past medical problems, and therapeutic treatments (such as chemotherapy or radiological therapy) as accurately as possible. This measure will not only save the client from needless repetition to other health professionals about when various events in his or her health history occurred but also enable you and other professionals to more easily retrieve old records.

Guideline 3

Use the client's own words, whenever possible, in recording symptoms or perceptions. Remember to put quotation marks around the client's exact words or statements. Recording direct quotations serves two important functions. First, it keeps the focus on the client's complaint, symptoms, or perceptions rather than on your interpretation of any remarks. Thus, it is a valuable primary source for other professionals who review the clinical record. Second, recording the client's own words prevents you from prematurely labeling his or her status until you have thoroughly assessed the situation by collecting more data or until you have carefully analyzed all the data to formulate a nursing diagnosis.

Guideline 4

Record, whenever possible, the chief complaint (or reason for contact or admission) in the client's own words. The chief complaint should be a brief, specific phrase stating the client's reason for seeking professional health care. The duration of the complaint is also included in the phrase. Examples of concisely stated chief complaints are

- Nausea and vomiting for past 2 days
- "Bad indigestion," 5 hours' duration
- Routine preemployment physical
- "Stomach cramps and diarrhea" since last Monday
- "I think I've got kidney trouble," 3 days' duration

Do not "translate" the chief complaint into a diagnosis, no matter how typical the complaint seems of a particular diagnosis. People rarely come to health care facilities with ready-made diagnoses. When a client tells you that "I've been vomiting bright red blood off and on for the past 2 hours," record the chief complaint rather than "ruptured esophageal varices" or "penetrating duodenal ulcer."

Guideline 5

Record under the heading "History of Current Illness" in a chronological narrative form, describing the onset of the complaint, its characteristics and frequency, its progress so far, and the reason for seeking help now. The letters PQRST can aid you in remembering to record the characteristics of the problem or symptom:

P—Provocative or palliative factors: those things that provoke or palliate the problem

Q—Quality: nature or character

R—Region: anatomical location

S—Severity: how the problem has affected the usual daily activities or lifestyle

T—Timing: duration of the problem

Generally, the section called "History of Current Illness" is the only part of the nursing assessment that needs to be written in narrative form, that is, in complete sentences and with appropriate paragraphing to permit the full sequential analysis of the problem.

Here is an example of a succinctly written history of current illness:

> Ten days ago Ms. V. O. noticed the gradual onset of midepigastric pain 2 hr after eating dinner. The pain has increased in regularity, however, so that it now occurs daily about 2–3 hr after every meal. She has also awakened for the past 3 nights around midnight with the same "burning pain"; it is relieved within an hour

after she drinks a glass of milk; then she can go back to sleep. This recent pain at night has "scared" her and caused her to seek medical attention. She believes that the "steady burning pain" is brought on after eating out at "fast-food restaurants," something she frequently does because of her job as a computer sales representative. Self-prescribed liquid and tablet antacids give her only "partial relief."

Guideline 6

Underline headings and indent the body of information if you record on an open assessment guide.[11] These measures make it easier for other professionals to follow your assessment. Consider the following portion of a nursing assessment in which *subj.* indicates subjective data and *obj.* indicates objective data:

Skin/Hygiene: (subj.) Showers b.i.d.—in morning "to wake up" and in evening "to perk myself up before studying." Has "a neurodermatitis" on both hands and neck in the winter, which causes intense itching, scaling, and crusting. Uses an external cortisone preparation ("I can't remember its name") given to her by Dr. E. 1 yr ago that usually relieves crusting. Denies pruritus and rashes at other times of year.
(obj.) Skin on hands shows evidence of lichenification; several 2–4 mm crusts on MCP joints (L) hand.
Sleep/Rest: (subj.) Sleeps about 5–6 hr a night during week; gets about 8 hr during weekend by sleeping later and/or napping.
(obj.) Yawning throughout interview.

Guideline 7

Distinguish between subjective data (what the client tells you) and objective data (what you observe, measure, inspect, or palpate) when you record your assessment, as shown in the previous guideline. Keeping the sources of data separate facilitates the assessment process and clarifies your findings to other professionals.

Guideline 8

Use the blank spaces on structured checklists as effectively as possible. Ellen Thomas Eggland recommends the following measures:

1. Use an *x* in the space to indicate the presence of a symptom.
   Example: palpitations __x__
2. Use a blank to write in specific information.
   Example: home diet __1,800 calories A.D.A.__
3. Use *no, none,* a dash (—), or leave the space blank to indicate that the symptom or item does not apply.[12]

Guideline 9
Use the comments section or blank space at the end of structured checklists to elaborate on the presence or absence of important symptoms or problems. If there is not enough space to complete your comments, state where they will be continued: "See nursing progress record for 8/13."

Guideline 10
Avoid the terms *negative, normal,* or *no difficulties* in the section "Review of Systems and Health Status." Instead, document specifically what is negative or what the client denies or has no difficulties with. This practice will inform other nurses and health care providers of just what questions you have asked, as shown below:

Respiratory: (subj.) Gets "one bad cold a year, usually every spring." Otherwise, negative for dyspnea, wheezing, cough. Denies bronchitis, pneumonia, asthma, tuberculosis.
(obj.) Breath sounds clear anteriorly and posteriorly.

Nursing Diagnoses

The nursing diagnosis is the end product of the assessment phase and of the written nursing assessment. Although definitions vary, it is usually viewed as a clear, concise statement describing the client's actual or potential health problems and based on nursing judgment after gathering and analyzing the appropriate data. In "Nursing Diagnoses and the Diagnostic Process," Marjory Gordon interprets nursing diagnoses as "health problems in which the responsibility for therapeutic decisions can be assumed by a professional nurse."[13] In "Nursing Diagnosis: Making a Concept Come Alive," Mary Radatovich Price states that a nursing diagnosis "identifies an existing or potential health problem that nurses are qualified and licensed to treat."[14] The nurse's role in formulating nursing diagnoses implies professional responsibility, educational qualifications, and state-sanctioned licensure. The health problems that nurses have the responsibility, capability, and licensure to treat are, in Gordon's words, "potential or actual disturbances in life processes, patterns, functions, or development, including those occurring secondary to disease."[15]

At the 1973, 1975, and 1978 National Conference on Classification of Nursing Diagnoses, 37 broad diagnostic categories that nurses can use to describe potential or actual health problems were accepted. Altered levels of consciousness, grieving, lack of knowledge, noncompliance, sensory-perceptual alteration, impaired thought processes, potential for trauma, and social isolation are some of the areas listed.[16] But because the categories are broad, it is imperative that nurses individualize each diagnosis to reflect the specific health problem. For instance, instead of writing just "noncompliance" for the man who refuses to take his cardiac medications, you could more profitably state: "noncompliance with cardiac medication regimen."

In formulating the nursing diagnosis, you must have sufficient data to suggest the appearance of a diagnostic pattern. Isolated cues, signs, or symptoms constitute insufficient evidence on which to base a diagnosis. Frequently, the nurse will have gathered enough information during the nursing assessment to be able to form a diagnosis. But sometimes sufficient data for a diagnosis do not become evident until several days after the client's admission to an acute care agency or until after several visits to an outpatient facility. Therefore, data collection via the initial nursing assessment and the continuous process of assessment/reassessment are crucial in writing an appropriate nursing diagnosis.

According to Gordon, the nursing diagnosis consists of three components: (1) "the state-of-the-patient" or health problem, (2) the etiology of the problem, and (3) the signs and symptoms.[17] This division has often been referred to as the PES (problem, etiology, signs and symptoms) format and is a convenient way in which to structure a nursing diagnosis. The problem component requires a clear, concise statement of the client's actual or potential health problem. The problem may originate from a combination of factors—psychological, sociological, physiological, environmental, cultural, or spiritual. As Gordon points out, "differentiation among possible etiologies is extremely important because each may require different therapy."[18] The third component, the signs and symptoms, constitutes the specific behavioral parameters used to make the diagnosis.

With the PES format, the nurse can prepare a nursing diagnosis in a systematic way and at the same time communicate effectively by permitting other professionals to share in the findings. Below are nursing diagnoses developed for two different clients. Notice that the broad diagnostic category appears first, followed by the subdiagnostic category or necessary qualification of the problem.

- *Client 1:* Mr. D. Craft is a 42-year-old self-employed optician.

  Problem: Alteration in comfort—lumbosacral pain.

  Etiology: Impaired body alignment; lack of knowledge about good body mechanics.

  Signs and Symptoms: Restless, changes position in bed slowly and with great difficulty. Grimaces whenever changing position. Not able to sit up straight in chair. Uses heating pad when in bed. Says frequently that his back hurts. Asks for p.r.n. pain med. q. 3–4 hr.

- *Client 2:* Mrs. B. Singleton, a 54-year-old part-time librarian, has recently had a cerebral hematoma.

  Problem: Sensory-perceptual alteration—misperception of environment.

  Etiology: Visual field disturbances.

  Signs and Symptoms: Cannot recognize common objects (dinnerware, cups, eyeglasses), unable to recognize family, does not recognize self in mirror. Unable to tell right from left, up from down, inside from outside.

Another way to write a nursing diagnosis, as reviewed by Mary O'Neil Mundinger and Grace Dotterer Jauron in their 1975 *Nursing Outlook* article, is to use a two-part nursing diagnosis statement. The statement is not a complete sentence; instead, it has two segments joined by *related to*. The first segment gives the health problem or the client's "unhealthful response."[19] The second segment supplies possible etiological factors. Some examples of this two-part statement method developed by Mundinger and Jauron are (1) "inadequate fluid intake related to lethargy and pyrexia," (2) "red sacrum related to inadequate circulation," and (3) "inadequate rest related to excessive TV noise in room."[20] You can see that the broad diagnostic categories used in the PES format do not appear here. However, "red sacrum" could be considered a subdiagnostic category of the broader "impairment of skin integrity" category; "inadequate fluid intake" is a subcategory of the broader "fluid volume deficit"; "inadequate rest" is another way of saying "dysrhythm of sleep-rest activity."

The selection of the phrase *related to* rather than *due to* reduces the chances of unlikely, but possible, legal complications. *Due to* implies a causal relationship, whereas *related to* specifies a relationship not necessarily linked to causative factors.

Just as Gordon and Price believe that appropriate nursing interventions result from the correct identification of the etiology of the problem in the PES format, Mundinger and Jauron also believe that the "related to" factors pinpoint the areas for specific nursing interventions.

And so the formulation of the nursing diagnosis is the result of data gathered during the initial nursing assessment and of continuous assessment/reassessment. As you will see in the next section, the nursing diagnosis is the basis for effective care planning.

CARE PLANS

A care plan is a summary or an outline of data about specific client problems, organized in a succinct, systematic manner. The plan promotes optimal care by stating the client's unique problems, the nurse's and the client's mutually agreed-upon goals to resolve those problems, and the specific interventions that the nurse and the client perform to attain the goals. The care plan functions as a guide for directing nursing actions toward the realization of the client's health care needs. The care plan, then, is an organized, systematic guide to goal-directed nursing care. Evaluation, an integral part of the care plan, ensures that the plan changes whenever necessary to meet the client's dynamic biopsychosocial status.

Clearly, the care plan consists of the written results of the nursing process. Through the documentation process, nurses can analyze the care regimen for the client and evaluate the entire plan of care or any of the elements of the care plan. The care plan documentation process has a dual purpose: (1) It provides a written plan for consistent, ordered, and continuous care. (2) The writing process assists the professional nurse in thinking more critically and analytically. Carefully thought-out problems, goals, and interventions give direction, specificity, and purpose to the nurse who is planning and delivering the care. No longer is care given in a vacuum without considering the client's unique biopsychosocial problems.

Importance of Care Plans

Care plans are important for several reasons. Nursing researcher Rudy L. Ciuca points out their value in the intraagency transfer of clients from areas of specialized care to those of less acute care, in the interagency transfer of clients from an acute care setting to a rehabilitation facility, and in the multidisciplinary approach to caring for the client. Since these three factors have the potential to disrupt the continuity of care, the importance of using a care plan becomes evident. Ciuca traces the care plan's development through three stages: "a means of communication, a professional assessment and diagnostic tool, and incorporation of a multidisciplinary approach." Yet Ciuca adds that, even as he writes his 1972 article, "these concepts are not reflected in actual practice."[21]

But the communication value of the care plan should not be underestimated. In fact, it is probably the primary communication tool at the nurse's disposal. "Written care plans form the foundation for the methodical communication of important elements in each client's nursing care,"[22] argue more recent researchers. Care plans can communicate to the nurse who wrote them, the nurse's colleagues, various team members, the client, the client's physician and family, and nurses on other units or in subsequent admissions, among others.

Components of Care Plans

Just as the nursing assessment supplies the data base for formulating the nursing diagnosis, so now does the nursing diagnosis provide the basis for initiating the plan of care. The three major components of the care plan are (1) the nursing diagnosis or problem, (2) long- and short-term goals, and (3) nursing orders. Some care plan formats (such as the one in Exhibit 2.3) include an evaluation column to remind the nurse that the evaluation phase of the nursing care planning process should be documented just like the other phases.

The nursing diagnosis furnishes the framework for identifying existing or potential problems and for developing client-centered goals that will be mutually agreeable to the client and the nurse. A problem is a deficit or potential deficit in the client's health status that is believed to need correction or that causes concern to the client or those caring for the client. Client-centered goals are frequently referred to as behavioral or "expected" outcomes.[23] Goals are usually stated in broad, general, nonmeasurable terms to identify effective criteria for evaluating nursing action. They may pertain to rehabilitation, prevention of complications associated with stressors, and/or the ability of the client to adapt to stressors.

Goals may be immediate and intermediate (short-term) or long-term. Long-term goals, synonymous with the nonquantifiable outcomes that

DATE	PROBLEM/NSG. DX.	DATE	LONG & SHORT TERM GOALS	DATE	NSG. ORDERS INTERVENTION	DATE	EVALUATION MODIFICATION
RM.#	NAME			AGE	RELIGION DOCTOR		

Exhibit 2.3. Nursing care plan that includes an evaluation column.

Professors Bailey and Claus describe,[24] are expected outcomes that describe the client's predicted behavior during the rehabilitation phase of his or her illness or during the resolution of his or her problem. Long-term goals may or may not be attained before a client is discharged from an agency. An illustration of a long-term goal for an 18-year-old woman with a nursing diagnosis of "alteration in nutrition—less than body requirement" might be, "Ms. H. T. will gain 2 lb per week until she weighs 100 lb."

Short-term goals, on the other hand, are expected outcomes that describe the client's predicted behavior during the acute phase of the illness. They should be derived from long-term goals, be achieved during a specified time, be ranked according to priority, and be modified as necessary. For Ms. H. T., appropriate short-term goals could be

1. Will eat all food on tray at mealtimes within 1 hr of being served
2. Will refrain from self-induced vomiting
3. Will drink milkshake H.S. within ½ hr of being served

The identification of the client's problem and the formulation of long- and short-term goals are prerequisites for nursing orders, or nurse-to-nurse directives on the management of client-centered care. Because nursing orders derive from the nursing diagnosis, they are "systematically designed to treat the cause of the client's health problem—in other words, to focus on the etiology."[25] Consider the following entry on a care plan:

Date	Problem	Goal	Nursing Orders
4/7			1. Force fluids to 3,000 cc per day.
			2. Offer 4 oz juice at 10 am, 2 pm, 7 pm

The difficulty with this notation is that we are writing well-known nursing orders in a prescriptive "cookbook" approach. We do not know the client's problem, nor do we know what the nurse's goals are for the client. By not defining these parameters, the nurse operates under prescriptions that may or may not fit the client's needs. By omitting the statement of the problem and the goals, the nurse informs other professionals that the steps of the nursing process have not been used to assess, interpret, and diagnose the problem, to plan long- and short-term goals to resolve the problem, and to implement specific nursing orders that will meet those goals. Evaluation of each phase of the process should take place, too.

In this next situation, however, nursing orders are well-integrated into the plan of care:

> Mr. M. J. R., a 44-year-old building maintenance supervisor, was admitted to the neuroorthopedic unit after suffering a fractured left femur in a construction accident. After Mr. R. was placed in balanced skeletal traction, his nurse did an in-depth assessment and determined a potential problem with decreased bowel function. Potential or probable problems, we know, are ones that clients run a high risk of incurring, and most people who are immobilized tend to become constipated. The goal for Mr. R., which the nurse determined after talking with him about the effects of immobility on bowel function, was for him to maintain, as much as possible, his normal evacuation pattern. Specific nursing orders to achieve this goal were determined after assessing his food preferences and his previous use of laxatives. In effect, the client had input into his care plan, and the nurse was able to validate it with him.

Here is the care plan that the nurse and Mr. R. developed:

Date	Problem	Goal	Nursing Orders
6/19	Potentially decreased bowel function related to immobility and greatly reduced activity level.	Mr. R. will have a soft formed stool every other day after breakfast (similar to evacuation pattern at home). Routine will be established by 6/24.	1. Provide increased fiber—whole-wheat bread at all meals, prune juice at breakfast, raw vegetables and salads at lunch and supper, fresh fruit (apple or pear only) H.S. *Dietary notified.* 2. Give stool softener every other night (odd) H.S. 3. Offer 1 or 2 glycerine suppositories in AM (even days) 30 min after breakfast, if Mr. R. does not have urge to evacuate. 4. Encourage Mr. R. to drink 2,500 cc a day.

You can see that the preceding four nursing orders give specificity and direction to the attainment of the goal. Nursing orders coordinate and organize nursing activities to help ensure that each client makes continuous progress toward better health. Most importantly, nursing orders must be clear, concise, and directly related to the identified goal and problem.

Location and Format of Care Plans

The location and format of care plans vary according to the agency's organizational needs and client population. Care plans may be arranged for groups of clients (for example, a team, a module, or the "case assignment" of a primary nurse) in a flip-chart system. Or they may be kept in a larger 8½ × 11-in. loose-leaf notebook, on a clipboad at the side of the bed, or in the chart. The actual system is not important as long as it adequately meets the facility's needs. One important consideration, however, is that the care plan be readily accessible to all nursing personnel caring for the client.

Care plans appear in many formats. Earlier, in Exhibit 2.3, we saw a four-column care plan that includes an evaluation column. Nurses at the institution where this plan is used specifically designed such a format to

CONDITION: Satisfactory Fair Serious Critical			Date of Admission:	
ALLERGIES			Time of Admission:	
Diet N.P.O.	ORDERS AND TREATMENTS		Date	NARCOTICS & P.R.N.s
Liq:	Vital Signs:			
Soft Regular				
Special:	Sitz Bath:			
Feed Assist Self				
I&O T.A.C.				
Force Restrict				
Tubes	In	Out		
Foley				
Levine				
Other				
			SPECIAL PROCEDURES	
L.B.M.			Clips/Sutures/Staples:	
DIAGNOSIS/OPERATION				
	Resp. Therapy		Pack:	
			Drains:	
	P.T.			
	PAP Smear: done refused		Consult:	
	To be done by Dr.			

Exhibit 2.4. Semistructured Cardex.

encourage the application of all four phases of the nursing process. The form opens up to provide additional writing space.

Other cards often grouped with the care plan include Cardex or Rand forms. These convenient worksheets contain information about diagnostic studies, medications, and treatments ordered by nurses or physicians (for example, intake and output, vital sign routines, type of bath, activity, and diet). Many of these items are arranged in a semistructured format that eases the work of the unit clerk who transcribes the orders and of the professional nurse who must employ ancillary personnel to assist in client care delivery (Exhibit 2.4).

Another type of Cardex form is a checklist based on the essential elements of the assessment phase of the nursing process (Exhibit 2.5). Here the nurse can quickly document the client's biopsychosocial status and related nursing care needs, and update them as necessary.

A Cardex may also be a combination of standard orders, care plan, and diagnostic/therapeutic worksheet. Exhibit 2.6 shows a care card for a coronary care unit with pertinent standing orders on the front. When the card is opened (Exhibit 2.7), the care plan and worksheet are visible.

Guidelines for Writing Care Plans

We recommend 12 guidelines to aid the professional in writing effective care plans. When you follow these suggestions, you can be more certain that the plan you devise will be successful.

Guideline 1
Before writing the initial care plan, review, assess, and analyze the appropriate input or the data base. Items that can provide significant information include

- The admission nursing assessment
- The admitting diagnosis
- The client's chief complaint or reason for admission (frequently different from the physician's admitting diagnosis)
- Initial or routine lab work
- Sociocultural status
- The medical history and physical exam
- Observations from other members of the health care team

Guideline 2
Always categorize problems as *actual, potential,* or *possible.* Note the date when problems were first identified. Actual problems are identified by

RM. # ___ NAME: ___ AGE: ___ RELIGION: ___ DOCTOR: ___

MENTAL STATUS:
___ Alert
___ Drowsy
___ Disoriented
___ Time
___ Place
___ Person
___ Lethargic
___ Semi-Comatose
___ Comatose

LOCOMOTION:
___ Walks
___ Brace ___
___ Prothesis ___
___ Cast ___
___ Splint ___
___ Cane
___ Quadcane
___ Crutches
___ Walker
___ Wheelchair
___ Portalift
___ Paralysis ___
___ Amputation

EMOTIONAL STATUS:
___ Cheerful
___ Anxious
___ Fearful
___ Depressed
___ Angry
___ Suicidal
___ Other ___

BOWEL:
___ Incontinent
___ Colostomy
___ Ileostomy
___ Special Care
___ Self
___ Assist
___ Total

BLADDER:
___ Incontinent
___ Ureterostomy
___ Foley Catheter
___ Leg Bag
___ Leg Strap
___ Tape
___ Special Care
___ Self
___ Assist
___ Total

HOME MEDICATIONS
___
___

SIGHT:
___ Glasses
___ Contact Lenses
___ Prosthesis
___ Cataract ___
___ Blind ___

HEARING:
___ Hard of Hearing ___
___ Hearing Aid ___
___ Deaf ___
___ Lip Reads

SPEECH:
___ Aphasic
___ Mute
___ Laryngectomy
___ Esophageal Speech
___ Tracheostomy
___ Other ___

MOUTH:
___ Partial Plate/Bridge
___ Dentures
___ Proper Fit
___ Broken Teeth
___ Edentulous
___ Gastrostomy
___ Special Care
___ Self
___ Assist
___ Total

POSITION AND COMFORT:
___ Turn q2 Hours
___ Back Care
___ Footboard
___ Bed Cradle
___ Sandbags
___ Traction
___ Trapeze
___ Air Pressure Mattress
___ Sheepskin
___ Heel Protectors
___ Elbow Protectors
___ Feedbag
___ R.O.M.E.
___ Cotton Mattress

ADL:	S	A	T
Hair			
Shampoo			
Nails			
Shave			
Bath			
Tub			
Shower			
Bed			
Dress			
Shoes			
Assistive			
Devices			

SKIN:
___ Cyanosis
___ Erythema
___ Pallor
___ Jaundice
___ Ulceration
___ Excoriation
___ Abrasion
___ Laceration
___ Ecchymosis
___ Rash
___ Edema
___ Dryness
___ Oiliness

SAFETY:
___ Posey
___ Siderails
___ Soft Restraints
___ Bed in low position
___ Seizure Precaution
___ Security Room

RESOURCES:
SS ___
PT ___
OT ___
Resp. Ther. ___
VNS ___
Speech Ther. ___
Diet Ther. ___
Other ___

Exhibit 2.5. Cardex checklist assessment.

CORONARY CARE NURSING CARDEX   2665 (1-80)

Date

____ 1. Start "KO" I.V. 500cc 5% G/W — Use plastic needle, or #19 scalp vein needle.

____ 2. Should signs of clinical shock occur: start 250cc 5% G/W with Aramine 100 mgm, to maintain systolic pressure of 90-110. Notify Physician.

____ 3. Should PVC's occur 6 or more per min., or if multifocal in nature, run 2-3 together, or occur on the "T" wave — give Lidocaine 75 mgm bolus. If no response — Lidocaine 100 mgm every 5 min. x 2. Start 500cc 5% G/W with Lidocaine 1000 mgm and titrate to control PVC's — Notify Physician - Do not exceed 4 mgm/min.

____ 4. Should sinus bradycardia occur under rate 50, and symptomatic, give Atropine 0.6 mgm I.V. STAT and repeat in 10 min. if needed. Notify Physician.

____ 5. (a) Should 2nd. or 3rd. degree AV block occur with apical rate of 50 or below, give Atropine 0.6 mgm IV STAT, and repeat in 10 minutes if needed and Solu-Cortef 250 mgm IV. Notify Physician. If Atropine is ineffective, start Isuprel 1 mgm in 250cc 5% G/W and titrate intravenous to avoid PVC's and increase ventricular rate of 50-60/minute.
(b) Should 2nd. or 3rd. degree AV block occur and apical rate is above 50, Notify Physician before administering the Atropine or Solu Cortef.

____ 6. In the event of pulmonary edema apply rotating tourniquets as indicated, observing the peripheral circulation of legs at frequent intervals. — Notify Physician.

____ 7. Should ventricular fibrillation occur or ventricular tachycardia occur and the patient is moribund: nurse may administer precordial shock at 400 watt seconds and repeat 3-4 times. "DR. HEART" page should be placed immediately.

____ 8. Nurse may initiate cardiac resuscitation measures as indicated.

____ 9. Blood gases and Electrolytes STAT post cardiac arrest.

____ 10. Triglycerides to be done when I.V. is discontinued.

Exhibit 2.6. Coronary care Cardex (front).

Name:		Previous Hospitalization		
Emergency Phone Number				
1.		Orientation to CCU		
2.		Patient		Family

Diagnosis - as told by physician

Patient's Reaction

Date

Initial Introduction of Dx, Px, Rx

Goals-

CONDITION: Satisfactory Fair Serious   Date & time of admission:

Date & time of transfer:

DIET:	DAT	ORDERS AND TREATMENTS	Date	NARCOTICS & P.R.N.s
NPO		Vital Signs:		
Cl. liq.	Fl. liq.			
Soft	Regular	Sitz Bath:		
Special:		Cath.:		
		Monitor·		
Feed Assist.	Self			
I&O	T.A.C.			
Force	Restrict			
Bedrest	BSC BRP			
Dangle	Chair			
Up				
Self	Assist			SPECIAL PROCEDURES
L.B.M.		Resp. Therapy: Nasal O2		Clips/Sutures/Staples:
	DIAGNOSIS/OPERATION			CVP:
				Arterial Line:
		P.T.		Pacemaker:
				Others:
		PAP Smear: done refused		Consult:
		To be done by Dr.:		
RM. #:	NAME:		AGE: RELIGION:	DOCTOR:

Exhibit 2.7. Coronary care Cardex (back).

the nurse as being present at the time the assessment is made. Potential problems are ones that are likely to develop if preventive measures are not taken immediately. Because clients with indwelling Foley catheters run the risk of acquiring urinary tract infections (UTIs), these persons are often classified as having potential UTIs related to the presence of indwelling urinary catheters. Possible problems usually require the professional to collect more data before they can be identified or ruled out. On the care plan, you should preface potential and possible problems with the words *potential* and *possible*. However, the term *actual* does not precede actual problems.[26] All problems not labeled *potential* or *possible* are presumed to be actual, existing problems.

After writing your client's problems, ask yourself these questions:

- Are the problems phrased as clearly and concisely as possible?
- Do the problems reflect the subjective and objective data I've collected and reviewed?
- Do other professionals understand what I've written?
- Have I attempted to give the cause or etiology of each problem?
- Have I prefaced potential and possible problems with the terms *potential* and *possible*?
- Have I dated each problem?

Guideline 3
Use drawings and other graphic illustrations, whenever appropriate, to make the care plan more readily understandable. The case study below exemplifies this point:

> Mrs. B. F., a 56-year-old woman, underwent transverse colostomy surgery to relieve a bowel obstruction and to permit the distal portion of the bowel to heal. The proximal stoma was the functional opening leading to the upper bowel, whereas the distal stoma led to the nonfunctioning lower bowel. It was sometimes confusing for the nurses to remember which stoma to irrigate, until one creative nurse who was assigned to Mrs. B. F. decided to draw a diagram of the stomas right on the care plan:

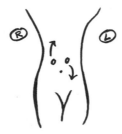

Under this freehand sketch, the nurse added the shorthand notation:

(R) stoma—proximal—IRRIGATE!

(L) stoma—distal—DO *NOT* IRRIGATE!

This combination of the drawing plus the relevant notation quickly clarified the nursing staff's responsibilities in irrigating Mrs. B. F.'s colostomy.

Guideline 4

Whenever possible, use only standard, acceptable abbreviations as listed in the American Hospital Association's recent publication, *Medical Record Departments in Hospitals: Guide to Organization.* That list gives you pharmacological, medical, and nursing abbreviations that are free from ambiguity.[27] (Although the poet's stock in trade is ambiguity, the professional nurse—for obvious reasons—strives to communicate one clear meaning.)

Frequently, however, agencies, physicians, and other ancillary medical personnel use nonstandard abbreviations that cause a great deal of frustration and uncertainty for the nurse who must decipher them. Although *"PT"* may be an acceptable abbreviation within one agency for *physical therapy,* there is always the danger that it could be confused with *prothrombin time.* More difficulties can occur when nonstandard abbreviations could easily be misconstrued. *PAT* on an obstetrical unit might signify "pregnancy at term," but it might also refer to a client's "paroxysmal atrial tachycardia" resulting from the stress of labor. In short, if it is common practice in your agency to use nonstandard abbreviations, be sure to make an up-to-date list available to all nursing, medical, and paramedical personnel. Avoid abbreviations whenever their use causes confusion.

Guideline 5

Write clear, specific goals that relate to the identified problems. Ask yourself—and the client when possible—what you expect that person to know, perform, or achieve by a given target date.

By way of illustration, let's review on page 63 some long- and short-term goals for Mrs. Georga Tempel, age 34, recently hospitalized when it was discovered that oral hypoglycemics, weight control, and diet therapy were no longer successful in managing her adult-onset diabetes mellitus. Ms. Pam Martin, the primary nurse assigned to Mrs. Tempel, interviewed and assessed her client; together they agreed on one long-term goal that Mrs. Tempel felt was very important for her to achieve by her tentative discharge date, 1 week away. Four short-term goals (often called objectives) were formulated to help Mrs. Tempel and Ms. Martin achieve the long-term goal.

Guideline 6

Always date and sign your nursing orders. Since orders should be reviewed and evaluated within a specified period, a dated order is essential. Signing your nursing orders indicates that you, as a professional nurse, assume responsibility and accountability for the formulation of the orders. Signing orders also informs others who care for the client just who is responsible for directing the care.

Date	Problem	Goals
3/7	Altered self-concept—dependent on others to give daily insulin, related to lack of knowledge about insulin and insulin administration.	*Long-Term:* Mrs. T. will be independent in her ability to give her own insulin and demonstrate her knowledge of diabetes management, by discharge on 3/14. *Short-Term:* 1. Mrs. T. will demonstrate the ability to draw up the correct amount of insulin, by 3/9 PM. 2. Mrs. T. will demonstrate the ability to administer her own insulin, using aseptic technique, by 3/11 AM. 3. Mrs. T. will verbalize to H. Monch, R.N., the onset, peak, and duration of NPH insulin, the s/s of insulin reaction, and the measures to help reverse the reaction, by 3/12 AM. 4. Mrs. T. will demonstrate the ability to maintain a site-oriented chart accurately, by 3/13 AM.

Guideline 7

Begin nursing orders with an action verb, which, by its very nature, helps you be specific, clear, and concise. Examples of nursing orders beginning with action verbs demanding specific, measurable activities are as follows:

- *Record* vital signs q. shift.
- *Weigh* client daily after he has voided and before he has eaten breakfast.
- *Irrigate* wound b.i.d. c̄ 40 cc half-strength H_2O_2.
- *Pack* wound loosely c̄ ½"-width Iodoform gauze b.i.d.
- *Measure* abdominal girth around umbilicus q. AM.
- *Elevate* head of bed 45°.

Action verbs emphasizing teaching activities include

- *Instruct* Mr. S. in the use of blow bottles.
- *Inform* client of the reason for respiratory isolation.
- *Show* Mr. Z. how to do isometric exercises on 3/30.
- *Discuss* s/s of hypoglycemic reactions on 12/15 PM.
- *Demonstrate* tube-feeding procedure to Mr. J.'s wife.

- *Answer* questions and clarify misunderstandings about nature of hypertension.

Another type of action verb chosen by the nurse often refers to psychosocial skills:

- *Encourage* socializing with others in the dining room.
- *Reassure* client by helping her focus on her achievements.
- *Allow* Mr. P. to freely verbalize fears of impending surgery.
- *Maintain* a calm, unhurried appearance while in the room.

Guideline 8
Apply the principle of specificity in writing nursing orders. To be effective and complete, they should answer, as needed, such questions as *who, when, what, how much,* and *how long.*

- *Who?* This question is often addressed when someone with specialized skills (for example, a psychiatric clinical nurse specialist) will help care for the client or provide one aspect of that care. Or the primary nurse, after identifying a problem, may delegate to the associate nurse the interventions to resolve the problem.
  Examples: • Provide Mrs. R. c̄ information about where she can obtain colostomy equipment at the lowest possible price. (To be done by K. White, home care coordinator.)
  • Discuss client's perception of his illness and his long-range plans. (Delegated to N. Dangerfield, R.N.)
- *When?* All nurse-initiated treatments should specify the times they are to be performed. If the times are different from the agency's accepted definition of b.i.d., t.i.d., q.i.d., etc., this fact should be clearly indicated in the order. The time element also becomes important if it is associated with other nursing actions.
  Examples: • Instruct Mr. F. in the use of quadriceps-setting exercises during AM care on 4/4.
  • Give 4 oz fruit juice at midmorning (10–10:30AM) and at midafternoon (2–3 PM).
- *What?* This area has the greatest potential for not being specific when all the information is not included in the nursing order. What is the difference between the following examples?
  Examples: • Provide Mr. G. c̄ information about his x-ray.
  • Provide Mr. G. c̄ x-ray information sheet, "All About a Barium Enema."

- *How Much?* Quantity can be a necessary element in improving the specificity of your nursing orders. For the client whose calories or fluid intake must be restricted, detailing exact quantities can be crucial. Can you explain the difference between the following orders?

  Examples:　• Restrict fluid intake to 1,000 cc per day.
  　　　　　　• Restrict fluid intake to 1,000 cc each 24 hr: 500 cc, 7–3, 400 cc, 3–11, and 100 cc, 11–7. (Dietary will supply on tray 150 cc at breakfast, 200 cc at lunch, and 200 cc at dinner.)

- *How Long?* Seconds? Minutes? One hour or 2? The duration of many nursing activities can prove essential to their successful implementation.

  Examples:　• Use heat lamp to coccyx for 15 min b.i.d. at 10 AM and 7 PM.
  　　　　　　• Spend 15 min q. AM c̄ Mrs. O. to allow her to verbalize feelings about hospitalization.

Guideline 9

In certain situations, write a brief rationale with your nursing order so that your colleagues do not overlook the obvious. Then, too, a rationale may be helpful if others are not accustomed to working with the specific problems that the client has.

　　Example:　Use flowered sheets and colored blankets on Ms. V.'s bed. (All-white bed linen increases glare and visual distortion in the elderly.)

Guideline 10

Always write the care plan in ink and sign your name. Never use pencil. Because most agencies consider the plan a permanent part of the medical record, it deserves to be treated with respect. Never erase any portion of the plan or apply typewriter correction fluid to eradicate errors. Instead, try using a yellow highlighter to cross out resolved problems or problems for which the plan must be modified or revised. The highlighter has the advantage of reminding the professional what the previous plan of care was.

Guideline 11

Whenever possible, allow the client or family input into care planning so as to make the client a part of the planning process and to validate your perceptions of this client's problems.

Guideline 12

Review and/or update the care plan at least daily or more frequently, if necessary. This review should be done by the primary nurse or a nurse who has sufficient contact with the client to assess and evaluate fully this person's response to nursing care. Daily revision of the plan will prevent its becoming obsolete as the client's status changes.

TEACHING PLANS

Devising appropriate teaching activities is an essential part of the planning and implementation phases of the nursing process just as much as creating efficient, effective nursing care plans is. And in the last two decades, nurses have become more actively involved in formulating and writing teaching plans for clients with various acute or chronic health needs. In this section we present a historical perspective of the nurse's role in teaching health education, a rationale for planned instruction, a sample teaching plan format, 10 teaching guidelines with their implications for documentation, and ways to write meaningful instructional or performance objectives.

Historical Perspective

The teaching process has always been an integral part of modern nursing. British nurses of the late nineteenth century believed in the importance of teaching families about disease prevention, sanitation principles, and the care of sick family members. Florence Nightingale wrote extensively on problems in public health such as sanitation, public housing, and health teaching.[28] The example in public health education set by the English nurses no doubt helped pave the way for public health nurses to engage in health teaching to the indigent immigrant population in the United States. Indeed, health education of the public through programs on nutrition, sanitation, and maternal-child health has long been considered an accepted function of those engaged in public health.[29]

Ironically, while public health nurses were encouraged and expected to teach, nurses working in acute care institutions during the first half of the twentieth century were frequently thwarted in their attempts to establish planned teaching-learning experiences for their clients. Our analysis of *The Technic of Nursing,* a 1935 text by Minnie Goodnow, R.N., indicates that just about the only teaching the hospital nurse did was to dispense information about hospital rules when the client was admitted: "Tell her when she is likely to see a doctor, and explain about day and night nurses. Show her how to call a nurse."[30] Discharge teaching—"A mother may need instruction in regard to the care of her baby, the diet of an older child, or some special treatment to be given"[31]—was outside the hospital nurse's jurisdiction. Problems in health teaching such as these were channeled to Social Service. Interestingly, as early as 1918, the National League of Nursing Education issued statements that reflected a concern for educating nurses to assume teaching responsibilities toward their clients.[32]

During the past two decades, nurses have been able to become actively involved in client education, not only in ambulatory facilities but also in acute care and long-term care facilities. The reasons for this change are varied. First, we have seen a kind of philosophical shift in nursing from caring for clients with specific diseases to an increasing concern with helping people stay well. Nursing's concern with the client's altered state of wellness places emphasis on helping clients regain optimal health through appropriate health teaching. Another important factor that has greatly influenced health education is the consumer movement and the spiraling cost of health care. The difficulties that many families face when they are caught in the vise of inflation make it clear to them that it is much cheaper to stay healthy than to get sick.[33] Self-help books on various health topics, the proliferation of vitamins and health foods, and the growing desire to keep informed about one's own body have created an encouraging climate for establishing planned teaching and learning experiences for the hospitalized client or the client in the outpatient clinic.

Other developments that have reflected the growing interest in health education during the 1960s and 1970s include the funding by the United States Public Health Service of planned client and family education projects on several chronic diseases, the sponsorship by the American Medical Association of several conferences on health education, and the creation in 1971 of the President's Committee on Health Education. In 1972 the American Hospital Association adopted "A Patient's Bill of Rights." Moreover, 8 of these 12 rights deal with communication—with informing clients about some aspect of their care. Two years later, the National Association of Children's Hospitals and Related Institutions adopted its own client bill of rights. And the pediatric bill of rights developed at Los Angeles Children's Hospital explicitly treats health education in its third article: "I have the right to expect my Doctors and Nurses to teach me and my family all we need to know about my illness so we can help me to recover and to stay well." Other than the passage of specific legislation (such as the 1973 Health Maintenance Organization Act, which made HMOs responsible for providing health education to their clients), perhaps one of the most influential factors in the establishment of client education was the Blue Cross Association's 1975 publication, *White Paper on Health Education,* supporting third-party reimbursement for client education costs.[34]

Planned Instruction and Spontaneous Teaching

In light of the approval of many federal agencies, the demand of the public for the "right to know," and the backing of private health care agencies, it is now much more important than ever to plan, organize, and document client teaching experiences. Simply because nurses plan their teaching activities, however, does not mean they must relinquish spontaneous opportunities to teach their clients. By no means should you equate written teaching plans only with formal learning experiences. Spontaneous teaching experiences will always occur, and nurses will need to take advantage of these whenever they come up. Nurses who are familiar with planned teaching guides, who know what their clients' learning needs are, and who review their clients' learning progress are much better able to take advantage of these spontaneous opportunities when a client demonstrates his willingness to learn *now,* for example, what effect his myocardial infarction will have on his sexual relationship with his wife. As Laurel Ratcliff Talabere points out, there exists "a certain security in planned teaching because we are ready for it."[35] The security of planning gives teaching activities a firmer basis when we are able to use spontaneous time. In Margaret L. Pohl's view, *"teaching which is planned for . . . is more effective teaching."*[36] Clearly, planned teaching can occur informally (in casual conversation, by example, by asking and answering questions) or formally (through lectures, discussions, demonstrations); it can happen at prearranged times or spontaneously.

Ideally, nurses should write and use planned teaching-learning guides for all clients. As a methodological tool, the structured teaching guide assists the nurse in better meeting clients' learning needs and in helping clients master prerequisite skills or coping mechanisms to adapt to an altered health status.

How complex this planned teaching should be depends on the biopsychosocial status of the client. The 22-year-old newly married teacher who has had a colostomy as a result of Crohn's disease will have different teaching-learning needs from the 75-year-old man who has had a colostomy as a result of carcinoma of the sigmoid colon. Because we can predict with some degree of certainty that each person will adapt differently in the modes of physiological needs, self-concept, role function, and interdependence, their teaching-learning needs will be different. The ways in which each client adapts will give cues to the perceptive nurse on how to plan teaching activities.

Actually, the basic content of the teaching plan for both ostomy clients will be similar. As one client education authority aptly states, "Although the 'what' in patient teaching is easy, it is the 'how'—or the process of teaching—that is the critical key to the success or failure of such educational efforts."[37] You know *what* to teach ostomy clients, but just *how* do you go about this teaching process? There are many factors involved here, and we encourage you to check into some of the references or additional readings listed at the end of this chapter. From our point of view, the *how* of teaching can be greatly facilitated by using, critiquing, and learning to write selected teaching plans.

To help formalize the content of teaching plans, nurses at many agencies have, through interdisciplinary conferences, developed standard teaching plans that are then available as teaching resources for all nurses in the institution.[38] The benefits are many. For one thing, the medical staff is less likely to resist client education when it has had input into what clients are being taught about hypertension, hepatitis, or cast care. Nurses who float, work part-time, or cover several units are more likely to participate in teaching-learning activities when they are aware of the standard plans. And nurses who work on a specialized unit (such as orthopedics) are more comfortable about teaching clients how to manage problems they don't usually encounter on the unit (such as duodenal ulcer) when they have access to a standard teaching plan (as well as a resource person from a medical unit!).

Yet standard plans afford but a basic framework for nurses to build on in their teaching activities. Only a systematic assessment of the client's learning needs will tell you what other things your learner *wants* to know to meet self-esteem or role-function needs or *ought* to know to meet physiological needs. Standard plans should be sufficiently flexible to permit content to be identified that is not applicable to the client's situation. And there should be enough space to allow for expansion of the original teaching plan as further learning needs are identified.

Format Selection

There are several valuable formats one can use in writing teaching plans. "The major criterion in judging the format is whether it facilitates the relationships between its parts,"[39] notes Barbara Klug Redman. One point to recall when selecting a format is that the format gives structure, consistency, and cohesiveness to the process of planning teaching-learning activities and client-centered learning objectives. That format which best exemplifies this relationship among objectives, content, and learning activities is the one to use. Perhaps the most important consideration for many agencies is consistency. It is difficult to imagine, for instance, how the teaching plans and guides recently developed at Tufts–New England Medical Center Hospital could have been so successful, with so many nurse educators and nursing practitioners contributing to them, if the format had not been consistent. Using a consistent format in the teaching plan also permits nonnursing personnel to become more easily acquainted with the teaching plans.

Furthermore, the same format should be usable for "standard" teaching plans as well as for individual plans. Because standardized teaching plans necessarily state probable learning objectives and must be broad enough to suit most learners' needs, it is important to be able to easily adapt them for individual needs.

The teaching plan format shown in Exhibit 2.8 works for standardized plans or for planning strategies for people with unusual learning problems. It can also be adapted for formal group instruction (Exhibit 2.9).

Exhibit 2.8. Teaching plan with three columns.

TEACHING PLAN FOR _____

DATA
     TOPIC:
     LEARNER AUDIENCE:
     GOALS:

     INSTRUCTOR(S):   TIME: LOCATION:
     TEACHING METHODS:
     METHOD(S) OF EVALUATION:
     SPECIAL EQUIPMENT/MATERIALS:
     ADVANCE PREPARATION:

Objectives	Content	Teaching-Learning Activities

Exhibit 2.9. Teaching plan for formal group instruction on the Milwaukee brace.

TOPIC:	Introduction to the Milwaukee brace.
LEARNERS:	All newly diagnosed scoliosis clients attending the University Hospital Outpatient Department's Scoliosis Screening Clinic or those referred by participating physicians.
GOALS:	1. To prepare newly diagnosed scoliosis clients intellectually and psychologically for wearing the Milwaukee brace.
	2. To foster the formation of a peer reference group to offer each other support.
	3. To introduce clients to the support services of the scoliosis clinic nurses.
INSTRUCTORS:	R. Williams, R.N., and M. Tomasik, R.N.
TIME:	6:00 to 9:00 PM, second Tuesday of the month.
PLACE:	Room 430, North Wing, University Hospital Outpatient Classroom.
TEACHING METHODS:	Lecture-discussion, demonstration.
MATERIALS:	See below for special equipment.
PREPARATION:	Before each class:
	1. Notify all participants by phone or mail 1 week in advance.
	2. Requisition teaching aids (x-ray view box, 16-mm projector, Sally Skeleton) 3 – 4 days before class.
	3. Send dietary requisition for soft drinks, fruit, and cookies 2 days before class.
	4. Gather equipment and handouts for the meeting on the day of the class: flip charts, x-rays, film, posttests, pamphlets.

Time	Objectives	Content	Teaching-Learning Activities
15 min	Clients demonstrate attitude of decreased anxiety and minimal discomfort in group.	Introduction to session	Instructors introduce themselves. Give out their extensions at clinic. Clients introduce themselves.
15 min	Clients demonstrate knowledge of scoliosis by identifying all signs and symptoms from a written list on a posttest.	Signs and symptoms of scoliosis: •Asymmetrical scapulae •Spinal curve •Protruding hip •Uneven dress length	Lead group discussion. Ask learners what they know about scoliosis and what they would like to learn. Ask learners what they noticed in their bodies. Summarize findings.
30 min	Clients correctly define four out of six terms related to scoliosis in a multiple-choice format on posttest.	Terms related to scoliosis: •Kyphosis •Lordosis •Congenital •Spinal column •Vertebrae •Scapulae •Convexity •Concavity •Curvature	Introduce and discuss terms, one at a time, using flip chart, Sally Skeleton, and spinal column. Use x-ray films to show change from initial diagnosis of scoliosis to post-brace period. *Learners:* •Can touch and inspect vertebrae •Can trace or outline curves on x-rays films

Exhibit 2.9. (Continued)

30 min	Clients correctly identify on written posttest rationale for use of Milwaukee brace.	The Milwaukee brace	Discuss purpose of brace and what it will do. Instructor no. 1 helps no. 2 demonstrate putting brace on. Let clients touch, feel, explore brace. Encourage them to put it on, if they wish. Show 10-min film, "You and Your Milwaukee Brace."
10 min	Clients correctly identify, from a written list on a posttest, all the sports in which they may participate, wearing brace.	Participating in sports or school activities *Permitted:* Camping, fishing, swimming, volleyball, biking, golfing, tennis, hiking *Not Permitted:* Contact sports (football, basketball, horseback riding)	Ask learners what sports they enjoy. Emphasize that while swimming they won't wear the brace. Explain reason for not participating in horseback riding or contact sports.
20 min		Break	Tell learners where restrooms are. Offer refreshments.
30 min	On a written posttest clients identify correctly the daily measures to care for brace and skin.	Brace and skin care	Discussion-demonstration of washing brace and caring for skin: *Brace*—Use washcloth, soap, and water to wash. Rinse $\bar{c}$ clear water. Do not immerse brace. *Skin*—Remove brace for ½ hr q.d. Inspect skin for reddened areas. Use alcohol to toughen skin and cornstarch to absorb perspiration. Wear cotton undershirt under brace.
20 min	Clients will verbalize questions or concerns following the administration and discussion of posttest.	Posttest (10 min) and follow-up discussion (10 min)	Administer posttest. Discuss answers. Answer questions. Let learners keep test as source of information.
10 min	Clients will verbalize understanding of how to have further questions answered and how to contact scoliosis clinic nurses.	Availability of resource persons.	Distribute pamphlet, "You and the Scoliosis Clinic."

The three-column setup readily allows the nurse educator to remember the relationship between the objectives, content, and teaching-learning activities in writing the plan. Depending on the nature of the topic and the learner audience, it may not be necessary to complete all the data headings. And so the nurse who is going to teach the client on an individual basis about hypertension control needs no special equipment; nor does the educator, in this case, need to be concerned about establishing a specific time and location.

Guidelines for Writing Teaching Plans

The goal of any teaching plan is to help meet the client's *learning* needs. Obviously, teaching is ineffective if the desired learning has not taken place. Thus, it is essential that the teaching plan incorporate associated learning activities that will help the learner achieve the goals and objectives.

Many principles guide teaching and learning. Although we will not discuss them in detail here, we have adapted 10 teaching principles that Pohl, in her book *The Teaching Function of the Nursing Practitioner*, identifies as having special relevance for nurses in clinical settings.[40]* After each principle, we will discuss the implications for teaching plans.

1. *Your teaching activities will have a better chance for success if you have good rapport with your client.* No matter how well thought out and well written the teaching plan, learning will not be as effective if the relationship between the two people in this communication situation is not comfortable and cooperative. Rapport flourishes when both the nurse and the learner (whenever possible) mutually define learning goals.

2. *You need effective communication skills for successful teaching.* The thrust of *Effective Communication in Nursing* is the necessity of using and adapting appropriate communication skills in many situations. When nurses teach, they must frequently adapt, modify, or change their verbal or nonverbal behavior to meet their clients' learning needs. If the nurse discovers that certain terminology confuses clients, it is wise to write on the teaching plan what does work. For example, nurses at one institution found that many newly diagnosed diabetics had a difficult time understanding why urine testing was an important part of their care if the problem was too much sugar in their blood. When nurse educa-

---

*Adapted from Pohl, Margaret L., *The Teaching Function of the Nursing Practitioner*, 3d ed. © 1968, 1973, 1978 by Wm. C. Brown Company Publishers, Dubuque, Iowa. With permission.

tors determined that one simple explanation worked well with most clients and decreased confusion, they incorporated it into their written teaching plan as a "teaching point":

Objectives	Content	Teaching-Learning Activities
Answers all questions on urine testing correctly 2 days after initial discussion.	Relationship between blood sugar and sugar in urine.	Teaching Point: "You will have too much sugar in your blood if you eat too much or you forget to take your diabetes medication. The extra sugar in your blood will spill out into your urine. So this is why it is important for you to test your urine regularly."

3. When you work with different ethnic groups, you need to know about their cultural patterns to teach successfully. Nurses who work with Cuban-Americans, for instance, and who want to set up teaching plans for classes on diabetic exchange diets should learn about their usual dietary preference patterns. Clearly, the teaching plan must reflect this knowledge, perhaps by listing specific foods for the bread exchange or by converting commonly prepared foods (such as the Cuban meat, fruit, and rice dish called *picadillo*) into component bread, fruit, and meat exchanges.

4. You can enhance the teaching-learning process by assessing your clients' unique learning needs. Before nurses can formulate and write teaching plans, whether individual or standardized for a given population, they should assess their clients' learning needs. Of course, one good way to do this is to use the nursing assessment interview. Other possibilities include using a questionnaire or a skills inventory checklist. Exhibit 2.10 contains a skills inventory checklist that could be used for a previously diagnosed diabetic client to help determine learning needs.[41]

5. You can gain your clients' cooperation if you ask them to assess what they feel they need to learn. Frequently, clients may feel unsure about their skills or knowledge even though nurses judge them competent and skillful in their actions. But nurses may gain a higher degree of cooperation from their learners if they involve them in evaluating their skills or knowledge. A "comfort index," as shown in Exhibit 2.11, is one way of doing this. Clients are much more likely to express their comfort about a skill or a concept than to admit that they don't know what they perceive nurses think they should know! In effect, a comfort index preserves clients' psychological safety and permits them to save face by not having to admit that they lack knowledge. This comfort index is designed to assess

Exhibit 2.10. Skills inventory checklist. [Source: Lilah Harper, "Developing and Evaluating a Patient Education Program," in *Patient Education* (New York: National League for Nursing, 1976), p. 4. Reprinted with permission of the publisher.]

SKILLS INVENTORY: DIABETIC PATIENT ON INSULIN

	Has Never Done	Needs Review	Does Without Review
1. Accurately measures insulin in syringe			
2. Rotates sites of injection			
3. Does insulin injection correctly			
4. Tests own urine for sugar and acetone			
5. Chooses 3 meals from cafeteria menu and stays within calculated diet			
Etc.			

Exhibit 2.11. Comfort index.

DIABETIC COMFORT INDEX

Skill/Knowledge	Yes	Sometimes	No
1. I feel comfortable about drawing up my own insulin every day.			
2. I feel comfortable about rotating my injection sites.			
3. I feel comfortable about giving my own insulin every day.			
4. I feel comfortable about testing my urine for sugar and acetone.			
5. I feel comfortable about using the Diabetic Exchange Lists to plan my meals at home.			
6. I feel comfortable about taking care of my skin and feet.			
7. I feel comfortable about knowing what to do if I can't eat because I'm sick to my stomach.			

a long-term diabetic's basic knowledge, but it could be used as an evaluation tool with newly diagnosed diabetics to see what additional instruction or reinforcement they need. Notice that the index is written from an individual client's point of view and that it contains simple medical terminology so that all clients will understand the meaning.

6. *You should use objectives as criteria or standards to help plan and evaluate teaching-learning activities.* Objectives written in terms of what you and the client have together agreed on serve as the foundation for effective teaching plans. When they are precisely and clearly written, you, as teacher, will have a better idea of the content of the lesson, the most logical sequence to enhance learning opportunities for the client, and the teaching methods best employed. Well-written objectives may also help you determine if you meet the overall purpose of the teaching plan. Also, clients will feel that they are not learning randomly but that they are learning those things that will help them manage their disease or altered health status and give them control over their lives. Writing meaningful objectives will be discussed in more detail shortly.

7. *You need to consider the time element when planning teaching-learning activities.* Nurses preparing teaching plans for presentation to groups of clients with related learning needs must frequently determine the best time of day to hold sessions, the appropriate length of time for sessions to last, and the best division of time among the related activities.

Suppose you are to lead a monthly group composed of teenagers who have recently learned that they have scoliosis that has to be corrected by the Milwaukee brace. Your goals are to form a peer reference group among the five or so teenagers who will attend your meeting, to prepare them emotionally and intellectually for wearing the Milwaukee brace, and to introduce them to the support services of the scoliosis clinic nurses. After determining that you have eight objectives that will help you meet three goals, you decide that you require 3 hours to accomplish your goals. After surveying other teenagers who come to the outpatient scoliosis clinic, you learn that after-school activities often last until 4:30 PM. You also learn from reviewing the social profile of all the clinic's scoliosis clients that about 85% participate in at least one extracurricular activity. And so you decide to hold your monthly meetings from 6:00 PM to 9:00 PM on the second Tuesday of every month.

Your teaching plan might look something like the one in Exhibit 2.9. Notice, especially, the time spent on class preparation as well as the time frames for each content area.

8. *You can control the learning environment for more effective teaching.* Many sociometric studies show that interaction improves when learners are comfortable and seated in open or circular arrangements. In instances in which the instructor sees the sharing of group experiences as necessary to the success of the class, it might be helpful to note this on the

plan under teaching-learning activities. Or if a specific classroom, because of its ventilation, lighting, and overall comfort, is more conducive to small-group teaching, this point could appear on the plan under special needs or materials.

9. *You should apply learning principles appropriately.* Several scientifically validated learning principles apply in thinking about and writing effective teaching plans. The influence of reinforcement on learning is one of the most common.

If the pulmonary clinical nurse specialist teaches Mr. Fry, an asthmatic client, to breathe slowly and diaphragmatically during acute attacks, he may still not follow through with these purposely controlled breathing exercises if the staff nurse caring for him does not also reinforce the nurse specialist's original instruction. This illustration points up the importance of having the teaching plan available to all professional nursing personnel. Also, just because Mr. Fry was once instructed in diaphragmatic breathing exercises does not mean he will remember how to do them correctly in stressful situations. He will, depending on his abilities, need to

- Think about what breathing patterns he has used in past asthmatic attacks
- See diaphragmatic breathing demonstrated at least once
- Imitate the nurse educator's skill until he feels proficient
- Practice the new skill at intervals until he feels he has mastered it
- Have others "cue" him (or give him reinforcement) in using diaphragmatic breathing when he has an acute attack

In short, Mr. Fry's teaching plan might be written as shown in Exhibit 2.12, taking into account that the appropriate use of demonstration, problem solving, repetition, and reinforcement can all help him to become more proficient in the use of a new psychomotor skill.

10. *You should realize that evaluation is an essential part of teaching.* Evaluation, the assessment of the goals or expected outcomes of an activity, is an ongoing process. Just as it serves to review the progress that you and the client make toward problem resolution during the nursing process, so is it crucial in determining whether the teaching-learning goals have been attained during the teaching process.

Go back to Exhibit 2.12 to review the evaluation method section on Mr. Fry's plan. Although the two objectives are stated in clear, behavioral terms, and although we can evaluate fairly easily if Mr. Fry has met them, we cannot lose sight of our goal—to enable the client to have purposeful control over his breathing during acute asthmatic attacks. Hence, our final evaluation method is to see if Mr. Fry can *transfer* the breathing

Exhibit 2.12. Teaching plan, with reinforcement, on using diaphragmatic breathing during asthmatic attacks.

TOPIC:	The use of diaphragmatic breathing during asthmatic attacks.
LEARNER:	Asthmatic clients who experience at least one acute episode of respiratory distress per year or who are hospitalized during an acute attack.
GOAL:	The client will have purposeful control over breathing during asthmatic attacks.
EVALUATION METHOD:	Instruction will have been successful if the client demonstrates successful use of abdominal breathing during an acute asthmatic attack. *Successful* use means no more than one initial reminder by the nurse when the attack begins and no more than two reminders to continue breathing exercises. Subjective evidence of success is the verbalization by the learner, up to 1 day after the acute asthmatic episode, that the exercises "help" during an attack.

Objectives	Content	Teaching-Learning Activities
Client will correctly verbalize to the clinical nurse specialist or primary nurse, 1 day after initial instruction, the main purpose in using diaphragmatic breathing during an asthmatic attack.	Rationale for using diaphragmatic breathing.	Assess past experiences: •How has client felt during other attacks? •Has anyone ever told client what to do during an attack? Has it worked? •Has client ever discovered anything on his own? Explain purpose of diaphragmatic breathing: "You won't feel as short of breath and as anxious because you'll be using your stomach muscles. Using your stomach muscles takes less energy and helps you breathe better during an attack."
Client will correctly demonstrate to the clinical nurse specialist or primary nurse, 2 days after initial instruction, abdominal breathing exercises for at least 3 full minutes.	Explanation/ demonstration of diaphragmatic breathing: •Sit slightly forward with hands on side of bed. •Place one hand over abdomen. •During expiration, push in and up on abdomen (diaphragm will go up). •Mentally picture slow, deep expiration. •Use no pressure on abdomen during inspiration.	1. Explain exercise to client. 2. Demonstrate exercise at least once. 3. Reinforce and correct behavior as client imitates the skill. 4. Give client sufficient time for practice and return demonstration. *Follow-up instruction:* Unit nurse checks client's understanding of exercises by asking client to demonstrate them at least once each day and evening after initial instructional session. Nurse reinforces or corrects behavior as necessary.

exercises he learned during the nonacute phase into purposeful, planned therapeutic activities during the attack phase. Should we find our clients unable to transfer learned skills to situations of greater seriousness, we may have to reconsider

- The entire teaching plan
- One aspect of the plan (such as, in this case, the goal of the client's having the ability to transfer skills from a stable environment to one of decreased stability)
- The methods for increasing and ensuring the ability to transfer skills

After careful evaluation we may, to cite one possibility, discover that reminding clients (or "cuing" them) to perform their breathing exercises is necessary *during* most acute attacks. So our plan may reflect this change by always including one family member in the teaching process.

Our five-part summary for writing successful teaching plans asks you to

1. Choose the best format to help you see the relationship between the objectives, content, and teaching-learning activities.
2. Write meaningful objectives that adequately reflect the behavior or knowledge you want your client to achieve.
3. Incorporate, when necessary, specific "teaching points" or you-attitude explanations to give to learners, to help them comprehend and achieve the objectives.
4. Employ brief phrases or statements to describe the content and the teaching-learning activities; complete sentences here are not usually necessary.
5. Prepare specific directions related to the content if the behavior to be achieved consists of several sequentially arranged items.

Writing Performance Objectives

Whether you write objectives as part of your client-centered nursing care plans or as a necessary component of your teaching plans, you should know how to state them clearly, coherently, and concisely. Measurable in terms of observable behavior, objectives may be considered the purpose, outcome, or product of an activity, implying a specific, well-conceived plan of action. They should be stated in terms of what learners "must be able to *do* or *perform* when they demonstrate mastery of the objective."[42] Performance objectives identify the measurable behavior or behavior patterns that will be accepted as evidence that the learner has achieved what we wanted him or her to achieve. Most importantly, they are learner-centered, not teacher-centered.

Some educational psychologists believe it more precise to refer to objectives as *terminal performances* since they refer to the end products of instruction.[43] Because objectives may be broad (such as those developed for an entire introductory course in microbiology) or very specific (such as those for a module on immunology), you will frequently see the terms *terminal performance objectives* and *interim performance objectives*.[44] The interim performance objectives deal with the attainment of more specific activities, usually accomplished within a smaller time frame. Psychologically, they are beneficial to the instructor and the learner, for they break down the terminal performance objective into smaller, well-defined steps. Definitive interim instructional objectives, arranged in sequence from the less complicated concepts to the more advanced concepts, greatly enhance the learner's progress and the logical plan of the instructor's teaching activities.

During the late 1940s, a group of psychologists and learning specialists spurred the development of objectives by identifying three different areas, or domains, of behavior. Benjamin S. Bloom and his colleagues identified these domains as cognitive, affective, and psychomotor. Cognitive behavioral objectives involve knowledge, mental ability, or intellectual skills. Affective objectives are concerned with the expression of feelings, values, attitudes, or appreciations. Psychomotor objectives imply what is commonly referred to as motor skills, physical dexterity, or manipulative behavior. A fourth domain, perceptual, has been proposed that deals with organizing and classifying shapes and patterns, including verbal and nonverbal meanings and images.[45]

Bloom and his co-workers further organized their domains into a taxonomic, hierarchical format. That is, the complex behaviors at the upper end of the taxonomy (numbered 5.0 or higher) included the less complicated behaviors (1.0) at the lower end of the scale. Exhibits 2.13, 2.14, and 2.15 diagram the domains in stair-stepped formations, illustrating that the lower numbers in a hierarchy must serve as the foundation for the next ordered concepts. Within the cognitive domain, for example, it is unreasonable to expect learners to compare two items (that is, apply the process of analysis) if they do not know how to describe them (that is, possess a basic knowledge of the items). Evaluation, the most complex behavior in the cognitive domain, depends on the five levels before it—synthesis, analysis, application, comprehension, and knowledge.

Writing meaningful behavioral objectives is not so difficult as it first may seem *if* you begin with an action verb that describes the specific interim or terminal performance or behavior you want your client to master, demonstrate, or achieve. You have to select the verb that best de-

Exhibit 2.13. The cognitive domain.

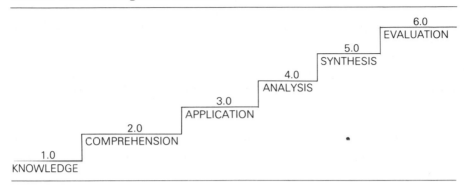

Exhibit 2.14. The affective domain.

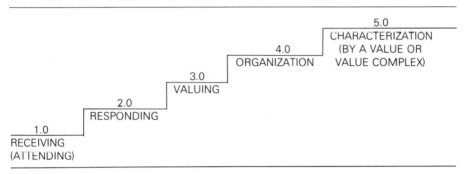

Exhibit 2.15. The psychomotor domain.

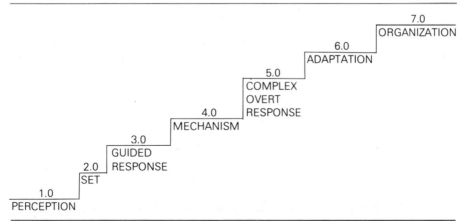

scribes the learning goal for your client since frequently the distinction between measurable and nonmeasurable objectives lies chiefly in the choice of the verb. The infinitive verb form is often used, for it saves time and prevents repetition. Verbs open to few interpretations in meaning give you the best handle on writing objectives. The italicized verbs below reflect the first level of the cognitive domain, have few interpretations, and generally will be easily understood by your learner:

- To *recall* 8 of the 10 risk factors associated with coronary artery disease
- To *record* urine test results for three consecutive days, using the diabetic flow record
- To *name* five county agencies that can help with resources for exceptional children
- To *define* the signs and symptoms of scoliosis
- To *list* seven symptoms of hypoglycemic reactions

Other verbs in the cognitive domain open to few interpretations appear next. As you read each one, try to determine at which level or levels the verb belongs (check your responses with Exhibit 2.16):

- To compare
- To classify
- To demonstrate
- To recognize
- To describe
- To apply
- To repeat
- To write
- To select
- To arrange
- To collect
- To inject
- To compile

Verbs open to several interpretations can create misunderstanding, confusion, or miscommunication on the part of either the teacher or the learner. Such verbs often evoke a subjective state such as thinking, feeling, or believing. You should try to avoid these terms since it is hard to measure them as manifestations of concrete, observable behavior:

- To grasp the significance of
- To internalize
- To appreciate
- To enjoy
- To feel
- To think
- To know
- To have faith in

Even though you have selected a specific action verb that tells the learner what you want him or her to do, be sure to determine whether the

Exhibit 2.16. Selected verbs to use in stating cognitive performance objectives.

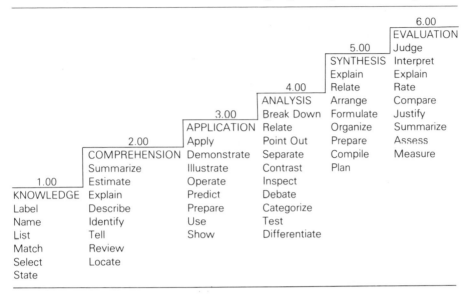

					6.00
					EVALUATION
				5.00	Judge
				SYNTHESIS	Interpret
				Explain	Explain
			4.00	Relate	Rate
			ANALYSIS	Arrange	Compare
		3.00	Break Down	Formulate	Justify
		APPLICATION	Relate	Organize	Summarize
	2.00	Apply	Point Out	Prepare	Assess
	COMPREHENSION	Demonstrate	Separate	Compile	Measure
	Summarize	Illustrate	Contrast	Plan	
1.00	Estimate	Operate	Inspect		
KNOWLEDGE	Explain	Predict	Debate		
Label	Describe	Prepare	Categorize		
Name	Identify	Use	Test		
List	Tell	Show	Differentiate		
Match	Review				
Select	Locate				
State					

learner's performance objective is stated overtly or covertly. In *Preparing Instructional Objectives,* Robert F. Mager uses the terms to describe performances that are directly observable (overt) or hidden (covert). Covert behaviors cannot be directly observed because they refer to performances that are internal, mental, or cognitive processes.[46] Suppose you decide you want your client to identify five signs and symptoms of a hypoglycemic reaction. But identifying is a covert skill, something that can be done mentally without a visually or audibly observable outcome. Just how do you expect the learner overtly to demonstrate the objective? By circling, underlining, writing, stating orally? Whenever the performance is stated covertly, be sure to clarify the objective by supplying an overt indicator, as in the statement, "Identify (write) five signs and symptoms of a hypoglycemic reaction."

Selecting the right verb helps you not only to clarify the performance you expect the learner to demonstrate as a result of the instruction but also to get a clearer picture of the lesson's content, the most logical sequence in which to present the lesson, and the most appropriate teaching methods to use. Generally speaking, people master simpler behaviors first, on their way to more complex ones. Assume you are writing a teaching plan to instruct a newly diagnosed diabetic on how to administer her insulin injections. If you analyze your objectives according to the verbs you have chosen, you will have a good idea of how meaningful your objectives are as well as whether they are in the most logical sequence for instruction (from the less complex to the more complex). For practice, analyze the following sequence of interim performance objectives. Which behavioral domains are involved? Does the sequence have a logical progression? Use the taxonomy in Exhibit 2.16 as your assessment tool.

1. To name the type of insulin she is taking
2. To describe the medication as it relates to
   a. Dose
   b. Onset, peak, duration of action
   c. Dietary restrictions or precautions
   d. Storage
3. To list the areas of the body where insulin can be given
4. To locate the outlines of these appropriate injection sites on her own body
5. To draw up exactly the correct dose of insulin
6. To demonstrate
   a. Cleansing the skin with alcohol
   b. Holding the syringe like a pencil
   c. Thrusting the needle quickly into the skin at a 90-degree angle
   d. Pulling back on the plunger to see if blood appears
   e. Injecting insulin at a steady rate over a 3 to 5-second period
   f. Withdrawing the needle quickly
   g. Placing an alcohol pad firmly on the injection site for 2 to 3 seconds
   h. Breaking off the needle on a disposable syringe

Although Mager explains that judiciously selecting the appropriate verb is paramount in the successful writing of objectives, he also holds that the important conditions under which learning occurs, together with the criteria necessary for acceptable performance, define the objective more precisely and make it more measurable.[47] Conditions imposed on the learner may include givens, restrictions, or allowances that clarify the learning environment and tell the client more about the situation in which he or she is expected to meet the objective. Here are some objectives containing specific conditions:

1. Given a copy of the agency's diabetic urine record, the learner will correctly record his a.c. and H.S. Ketodiastix results for three successive days.
2. Given a list of 20 foods, the learner will identify the 10 items high in sodium.

3. Given a diagram illustrating the anatomy of the femur and the acetabulum, the learner will correctly locate the site of her fracture.

Other "givens" that might be necessary as conditions of acceptable performance are models ("Given a model of the heart"), mannequins ("Demonstrate, through the use of the life-size infant training mannequin"), actual equipment ("Perform a colostomy irrigation using the Medex Co. ostomy irrigation set"), and specific sources of audiovisual information such as leaflets, pamphlets, books, or films ("Based on the booklet 'Breast Self-Examination,' list three ways to examine your breasts").

The criteria of acceptable performance make up the third quality of meaningful objectives. Here we are looking at standards by which to judge performance. The criteria should be expressed in a concrete, precise, and measurable manner, just as the performance itself is. Speed or time limit, accuracy or number, quality or acceptable deviation from the standard—these represent possible ways to describe the criteria of acceptable performance.

Review these objectives with criteria of various types:

- Completes posttest evaluation on hypertension within 2 weeks after attending classes.
- Draws up exact dose of daily insulin.
- Drinks no more than 1,050 cc nor less than 950 cc fluid daily.

In order to formulate well-written objectives, therefore, you should

1. Determine the specific performance that you want your learner to do, achieve, or master.
2. Decide in which category the performance belongs—cognitive, affective, or psychomotor.
3. Choose specific, measurable, concrete verbs open to few interpretations (rather than verbs open to many interpretations) that best describe the learner's performance activity.
4. State objectives in terms of future (*will* or *be able to*) expectations—what you want your learners to perform or demonstrate after a given class, practice session, or lecture-discussion.
5. Use the infinitive form of the verb to avoid repetition, especially with a series of objectives.
6. Include overt *(behavior indicator)* verbs whenever the performance must be translated into a directly observable activity.
7. Describe the conditions (givens or restrictions) under which the learner will be performing.

8. Add evaluation criteria or standards to pin down how well the learner must perform.
9. Arrange, whenever possible, series of objectives from the least complex performance behavior to the most complex performance behavior.
10. State just one specific performance for each objective; write as many objectives as necessary to communicate your overall performance goals.
11. Remember that complete objectives consist of three parts: performance, conditions, and criteria.

DOCUMENTATION SYSTEMS

In 1935 the nursing student who used Minnie Goodnow's *The Technic of Nursing* (then in its third edition, published by Saunders) studied four specific aspects of charting:

1. The graphing of temperature, pulse, and respiration
2. The graphing of weights
3. The maintenance of bedside records for all acutely ill patients
4. Detailed rules for printing clearly and rapidly

Indeed, as many pages were devoted to the mechanics of printing as to how and what to record on the bedside record. Students were taught to record "everything that you would tell the doctor, head nurse, or nurse who relieves you."[48] Goodnow's list of seven observations to be recorded (which she adapted from "Bellevue Nursing Procedures") included

1. Patient's symptoms, subjective and objective
2. Time at which everything occurs
3. Visits of physician and his orders
4. Treatments given
5. Patient's reaction to the treatment
6. Intake and output
7. Sleep and rest

A list of some 30 signs, symptoms, and treatments came next, to give the student further guidance in documentation. Her final point summarized how one should chart: "Records should be legible, grammatical, accurate, definite, logical, comprehensive, helpful to physician."[49] Today, surely, we would add "helpful to the nurse."

Although many of Goodnow's points about charting are still valid, there have been changes in the documentation process since 1935. Within the last two decades, the nurse's role in the documentation process has shifted its emphasis from recording solely the performance of specific therapeutic or maintenance activities and nonanalyzed signs and symptoms to recording analyses (nursing assessments and nursing diagnoses) and the process of nursing care planning.

Although the wide acceptance of the problem-oriented method of documentation and the application of the nursing process have undoubtedly made this shift possible, other reasons also account for this renewed interest in documentation. Because nursing is currently striving to establish itself as a distinct profession from that of medicine, the written documentation of nursing expertise, observations, analyses, plans, and standards becomes a very significant goal.[50] During the mid-1970s, the consumer movement greatly influenced trends in health care. And when the 1975 *White Paper on Health Education* supported third-party reimbursement for client education, nurses grew to realize that only specific documentation of their teaching plans and teaching activities would enable them to achieve professional and financial recognition.

What are your responsibilities as a nurse in documenting the care you plan, give, and evaluate? In their *Journal of Nursing Administration* article, Delores Thoma and Karen Pittman delineate three responsibilities of health care providers for documenting the care they give:

1. Responsibility to the patient to keep accurate, up-to-date records of services rendered and progress observed so that the care will be consistent with the patient's health needs.
2. Responsibility to the payment body to provide proof that such care was given, with observations of the results of such care.
3. Responsibilities of legal importance to provide a record reflecting care given and professional responsibilities for updating the skills and abilities of the health personnel through examination of their actions and judgment.[51]

Purpose and Content of the Clinical Record

All health agencies—physicians' offices, ambulatory care clinics, hospitals, nursing homes, health maintenance organizations, and visiting nurse associations—must keep clinical records on the clients for whom they render care or provide services. In effect, the clinical or medical record is a kind of business communication. Because the organization and maintenance of these records can be such a time-consuming and difficult task for those involved, consulting firms in systems analysis and information storage and retrieval have developed to help health care providers set up efficient record-keeping systems. Clinical record types, contents, and formats vary according to health agency needs. However, we can safely assume that facilities prefer records that are logically set up, readable, and understandable. The system itself should ease the retrieval of the clinical record.

Some of the purposes of the medical record listed by Mary D. Hemelt and Mary Ellen Mackert in their 1977 article for *Hospitals* include

- Providing a means of communication among health team members who are caring for the client
- Serving as a data base for planning individual care
- Serving as a data base for research or educational purposes
- Serving as a frame of reference for handling unexpected occurrences
- Supplying statistical data for public health and state planning agencies
- Providing data that the Joint Commission on Accreditation of Hospitals uses in evaluating health care agencies
- Furnishing documentation for clients involved in litigation, compensation, pensions, and insurance awards[52]

In addition, the record serves as a means of implementing nursing and medical audits, for it documents the client's condition at a given, specific time.

The components of the clinical record will reflect agency needs and client population. Usually, the contents reflect the physical and psychosocial assessment of the individual and his or her reaction to stressors, the plan of care initiated and implemented to resolve the client's problems, and the client's physical and emotional reaction to his or her illness or problems. Successful integration of the data should give a selective yet highly reliable profile of the client. The contents frequently incorporate the following items:

- Complete health history and physical examination, including the nursing admission assessment
- Physicians' orders and progress notes
- Nursing progress notes, nursing orders, and flow sheets to reflect activities of daily living, fluid balance, treatments, and vital signs

- Laboratory, radiological, and other noninvasive diagnostic data
- A progress record of treatments or therapeutic regimens performed by ancillary personnel
- Results of invasive or surgical procedures
- Client consent forms

General Documentation Guidelines

General documentation policies are developed to guide nurses as they work with and document on the clinical record. Although each agency has its own particular rules, the following eight guidelines are common to most health care institutions:

Guideline 1
Identify every page of the client's record with that person's full name, room number, admitting number, physician, and other identifying data. Often this information gets stamped on each page by means of a master plate and an imprinting machine.

Guideline 2
Write or print all entries legibly in ink. Do not erase any entry. If an error has been made (writing on the wrong chart or using the wrong word, for example), either circle or cross out neatly with one line the incorrect entry. Write *error* above the entry. Add your initials. Then immediately write the correct entry. Hemelt and Mackert (both are R.N.s, and Hemelt also holds a law degree) caution that erasures should never be permitted on medical records, for they raise questions and are "equivalent to telling a jury that one is hiding something."[53] They suggest that if an explanation for the error seems appropriate, the professional should include it. And for risky or complex situations, it might be best to have the corrected entry cosigned by another professional.

Guideline 3
Use quotation marks for anything clients say to describe their symptoms or feelings.

Guideline 4
Do not write *patient* or *client* in your recording since the entire record refers to the client. If there is a question about the meaning or clarity of an item, supply the client's name (Mr. Bowman) or initials (Mr. J. B.) so that there can be no misunderstanding.

Guideline 5
Note the date and time with every entry you make on the progress record
("4/4/82, 8:30 AM").

Guideline 6
Chart on every line, skipping no spaces between entries. Leave no blank
spaces on the record. Draw a line between the end of the entry and your
signature so that there are no spaces for others to make additions.

Guideline 7
Avoid indefinite phrases or terms such as *seems to be* and *appears*. These
two expressions, especially, add an element of value judgment or conjec-
ture to the documentation. As an illustration, an improper emergency
room notation for a client whose chief complaint is pain in the right forearm as a result of a fall from a 12-foot ladder would be: "Right arm appears to be broken." Instead, the more accurate, factual entry would read:
" 'Constant pain' (R) forearm, radiating from olecranon process to fingers.
Bruised area 4 cm × 2 cm ulnar aspect (R) forearm. No abrasions."

Guideline 8
Sign your first initial, last name, and status to every entry you make ("V.
Doti, R.N."). As a student, you will also need to add your school affiliation: L. Montgomery, S.N., K.S.U. (student nurse, Kent State University)
or P. Parker, U.A.N.S. (University of Akron nursing student). As a graduate nurse, you will find that many institutions prefer you not use
"G.N." since that is not recognized as an official title. In this case, you can
sign your first initial, last name, and the number on your state's interim
permit ("K. Cacciopo, #C6189").

The Source-oriented System

Basically, two types of documentation systems are available for recording
information on client records. First is the traditional source-oriented or
narrative system. Second is the problem-oriented system, developed by
Lawrence L. Weed, M.D., in the late 1960s. Both systems—or a combination of the two—are currently used and will be discussed.

In the source-oriented system, each health care provider writes on a
separate section of the chart, and the chart is divided according to who
originates the information. Nurse's notes are separate from physician's
orders and progress notes. Usually, dietitians, physical therapists,
respiratory therapists, and other ancillary personnel write on their own
progress forms. Notes are written in a narrative style, often with each
new item or separate topic put on a different line (Exhibit 2.17). The

			THE BARBERTON CITIZENS HOSPITAL NURSING PROGRESS RECORD
DATE	TIME	DATA	PERTINENT INFORMATION
5/16/81	12:30 Pm		Received from Recovery Room. Vital Signs upon return : BP 130/80 (R) arm, AP 88, respirations 20. Temp 99⁴ rectal. Skin warm and dry. Responding to verbal stimuli. IV of 1000 5% D/NS infusing at 20 gtts./min. ® forearm. Abdominal. dressing dry and intact. T-tube patent c̄ 50 cc. light green drainage in collection bag. NG (Salem Sump) to intermittent low suction draining dk. green.
	1 Pm		Assisted to cough and deep breathe. X 3. Turned to Ⓛ side.
	1³⁰Pm	Im meperidine	75 mg RUOQ for c/o incisional pain.
	2³⁰ Pm		Vital signs stable – see flow-sheet. Sleeping. Relief from pain obtained from Im med. Family at bedside L. Fox, RN
	4³⁰Pm		Assisted to turn, cough, and deep breathe. X 4. Lung clear to auscultation. Took few ice chips. NG patent. Voided 75 cc dk amber urine.
	5³⁰Pm	Im meperidine	75 mg LUOQ for c/o incisional pain.
	6³⁰ Pm		Restless: moving about in bed, moaning. No relief from Im med. given 1 hr. ago. BP up from previous readings (150/100 ®) – see flow sheet. Bladder dull to percussion. Unable to void when up c̄ assistance to bedside commode.
	6⁴⁵Pm		Physician contacted – order received to straight catheterize x 1.
	7 Pm		Catheterized c̄ No. 16 Fr. straight catheter : returns of 850 cc. dk amber urine in 10 min. Mrs. G. tolerated procedure well. Stated she felt "much better." — K. Nichols, RN

1094 (11-77)

Exhibit 2.17. Nursing progress entry (narrative style).

source-oriented documentation system follows a strict chronological order.

Since each health care provider writes in a separate section of the chart, it is often difficult to correlate the exact status of the client's progress, particularly if many members of the health care team are needed to plan and implement the client's care. This inherent difficulty in correlating the information recorded by health care providers on separate sections of the chart leads to unnecessary duplication of documentation.

Some critics of the source-oriented system view it as an obstacle to identifying client problems. The authors of *Problem-oriented Nursing* point out that in the traditional record, client problems and symptoms "do not appear in coherent order but are randomly scattered among other information which may be completely unevaluated and/or irrelevant."[54] Others see the source-oriented clinical record as perpetuating a system of "buried messages," that is, messages that only hint at client problems.[55] Buried messages about client problems may omit the full definition or identification of the problem, the implications, the nurse's recommendations, or the plan of nursing action. Buried messages, then, are also incomplete messages, lacking in comparative and qualitative judgments or assessments.

Writing in *Supervisor Nurse* about how and why nurses should improve the quality of their documentation, Aline MacDonnell Holmes isolates two further problems with the source-oriented documentation system. First, because nurse's notes and physician's notes are separated from each other, few physicians read nursing notes. This situation often results in nurse's notes that reflect tasks performed rather than observations of client behavior and condition. In addition, oral communication between nurse and physician tends to supplant written documentation. Yet while conversations between physician and nurse may be enjoyable and genial, they are also "an inaccurate and incomplete way of documenting care," and sometimes, concedes Holmes, they can "fail to communicate pertinent data in the presence of personality problems and the pressures of time."[56]

Guidelines for Narrative Recording

Even though the source-oriented or narrative system of charting does not provide the best means for communicating client care needs or problems, it can be used successfully if certain guidelines are followed.

Guideline 1
Review the physician's progress notes, the nurse's notes, and the progress notes from the other health care providers *before* you start charting. In this way, you can avoid unnecessarily duplicating information. And you may gain needed information about or insight into the client's problems.

Guideline 2
Take inventory of the client's status *before* you write. Ask yourself questions about this person's condition, problems, and progress. Has the condition changed under your care? How? Have new problems developed? If

so, document your subjective and objective observations, what measures you initiated to alleviate the problem, and the client's response. What about the progress or lack of progress made by the client toward resolving present problems?

Guideline 3
Remember, as a matter of general principle, to write nursing progress notes about

- A change in condition—whether physiological, behavioral, or emotional
- A lack of change in condition
- The development of new problems
- The resolution of old problems
- The response (behavioral and/or physiological) to treatments and medications
- The status of learning readiness
- The response to teaching-learning activities

Guideline 4
Summarize the client's biopsychosocial status whenever appropriate, especially in extended or long-term care facilities. Once the client adjusts to the facility, monthly summaries may be sufficient if new problems do not develop.[57] Some nursing homes chart on a different topic of nursing care each day of the week. This system can be especially effective in making certain that all the client's nursing care needs are regularly summarized.[58]

Guideline 5
Choose concise, clear phrases when you chart. Complete sentences are not necessary as long as you convey a single, clear meaning. If what you have written seems ambiguous, consult another professional for feedback on your entry.

Guideline 6
Use appropriate punctuation to clarify your intended meaning. In truth, punctuation "makes" sense. Evaluate the different meanings in these three entries:

1. Bathed in cardiac chair reading magazine.
2. Bathed. In cardiac chair, reading magazine.
3. Bathed in cardiac chair. Reading magazine.

Guideline 7
Be specific. Include necessary descriptions, measurements, and anatomical landmarks to communicate your message. "Abdominal girth 102 cm at umbilicus" conveys far more to the reader than "abdomen distended."

Guideline 8
If you write on more than one problem at a time, use separate paragraphs, to help keep the problems straight.

Guideline 9
Supply appropriate comparisons. For instance, if your client could walk the length of the hall today without becoming dyspneic, whereas yesterday she could walk only half the length of the hall, chart it this way:

> Improved ambulatory status as compared to yesterday. Today walked entire length of corridor s̄ becoming dyspneic. Respirations 20 and pulse steady and regular at 80 at end of activity. Yesterday could walk only half the length of the hall before becoming short of breath. _____ M. Gayetsky, R.N.

Guideline 10
Use graphic records and flow sheets appropriately and whenever possible, to help you eliminate extra documentation and avoid duplication of information.

The Problem-oriented System

The problem-oriented record system (PORS), the second method of documentation, is an effective tool that helps health care providers identify client problems; plan for their therapeutic, diagnostic, and educational management; evaluate and assess client progress; and summarize the course of the problems upon discharge.

The chief advantages of the PORS lie in two spheres: methodology and communication. Because the PORS emphasizes problem solving and the logical analysis of information, it is a system firmly based on scientific methodology. Because it furnishes one system of documentation for all professional health care providers and integrates *in sequence* information on client problems from nursing, medicine, social service, and other paramedical services, it is a more efficient communication system than the source-oriented record.

Like any tool, however, it is a means to an end—quality, comprehensive client-centered care. Since the use of the PORS has become so widespread in the past decade, we will discuss it here in some (although not exhaustive) detail.

By 1969, Dr. Lawrence L. Weed, then director of the outpatient department at Cleveland Metropolitan General Hospital and professor of medicine at Case Western Reserve University, had developed the PORS. As a medical researcher, he was struck by the so-called double standard in medicine, which still exists today. In other words, the physician-researcher follows strict guidelines, protocols, and rigorous discipline in pursuing the scientific methodology of problem solving when he or she defines a research problem. The physician-researcher continues with this discipline when preparing the manuscript detailing the results of the findings. On the other hand, the practitioner in clinical medicine abandons such discipline when faced with countless complex client problems. Since the documentation process that scientific methodology demands is often absent in clinical practice, progress notes and discharge summaries often fail to analyze the multiple physiological variables or to correlate them with psychosocial problems.[59]

The nature of the medical record itself was another factor that greatly influenced Weed's development of the PORS. In the traditional source-oriented record, the focus was not on the client's problems, needs, or complaints, but rather on who did what and when. Much too often, the chart became a "tangle of illogically assembled bits of information."[60] In complicated cases, it was almost impossible to trace the progress of various problems throughout the medical record. In fact, the chart frequently showed all too clearly just how unclear a practitioner's thinking was. Without the scientific methodology and without a tool to implement it, many problems were either not identified or else identified and treated less efficiently than they might have been.

The four basic components of the PORS are (1) data base, (2) problem list, (3) initial plans, and (4) progress notes. Since the nursing process employs the problem-solving method in client care, these two systems are quite compatible. Here is how the two systems interrelate:

Nursing Process	PORS
Assessment:	
Nursing history/Admission assessment	Data base
Nursing diagnosis	Problem list
Planning, Implementation	Initial plans
Evaluation	Progress notes

DATA BASE

The data base is an explicitly defined or predetermined standard baseline of information that is gathered about a client before his or her problems have been fully identified. The defined data base will usually depend on the setting; one for a client attending the pediatric well-baby clinic will be different from one established for adults attending the hypertension clinic. Certainly, the elements of the data base should be explicitly defined and meet the needs of the client population. In the *Guide to Patient Evaluation,* you can find nine elements that make up a rather complete data base for a hospitalized adult:

1. The chief complaint or reason for contact
2. History of present illness(es) or patient's perception of current health status if there is no illness present
3. Past health history
4. A logically arranged review of systems
5. Family health history
6. Personal/social history
7. Patient profile
8. Complete physical examination
9. Results of initial laboratory tests[61]

PROBLEM LIST

The problem list, in Weed's view, serves as a combined "table of contents" and "index" to the client's problems.[62] Just as the table of contents prefaces a book, so also the problem list appears as the first item on the clinical record. Problems are not necessarily diagnoses. They can be items that cause concern to the client or to those providing the client's care. Some common types of problems include (1) a specific diagnosis or syndrome, (2) signs or symptoms, (3) abnormal lab values, (4) allergies, (5) risk factors, (6) surgeries, (7) psychological problems, (8) social problems, and (9) demographic factors. Try to state problems at the highest level of resolution that the data will support. Naturally, previous experience and education will play a part here. The nurse practitioner, for instance, may identify three problems (pyrexia, myalgia, and productive, hacking cough) to the one problem (pneumonia) identified by the experienced diagnostician.

Many authorities who strictly adhere to Weed's original rules for establishing a PORS believe that all problems should be numbered. Attaching numbers to specific problems does not indicate a ranking or priority system but simply offers a shorthand means of identifying the problem. Once a number gets assigned to a problem, it always pertains exclusively to that problem. When a problem is resolved, its number never gets reassigned; instead, that number serves as a reference for the problem throughout the entire chart. Suppose, however, that while the problem in the problem list does not change, the statement of the problem changes.

What happens, then, to the number assigned to the problem? Consider the following example:

9/13 #1   Jaundice 9/18 Due to #5 Laennec's cirrhosis

9/13 #2   Hepatomegaly 9/18 Due to #5 Laennec's cirrhosis

9/13 #3   Decubitus ulcer (R) heel

9/15 #4   Allergic to codeine

9/18 #5   Laennec's cirrhosis

In this case, problems #1 and #2 were really manifestations of Laennec's cirrhosis. From 9/13 to 9/18, problems #1 and #2 were referred to in the clinical record as jaundice and hepatomegaly; but from 9/18 on, they will be included under problem #5, Laennec's cirrhosis. Notice how the dash and the date above it signal that the statement of the problem has changed.

As you might expect, some other professionals working extensively with the PORS believe that the numbering system is unnecessary, often unworkable, and rather awkward. In some people's minds, numbering problems from #1 on may be confused with setting up priorities of care. And accumulating numbered problems over several years can lead to some very complicated and perhaps perplexing problem lists. The decision whether or not to number might best be made by following the preference of the health care providers in the individual agency.

Once problems are resolved, they are transferred from the active column to the inactive column. Weed argues in favor of complete problem lists of active and inactive problems so that no previous significant difficulties (such as cholecystitis) will be overlooked if they recur or lead to complications. Others prefer to list at the front of the chart only those important problems that require attention at present.[63] In this scheme, inactive problems can be identified in the data base and in the progress notes, and they can be brought forward when necessary. Mixing in old, inactive, resolved problems with present problems may create too much noise in the system's information-processing channels.

The problem list, therefore, serves as a checklist of the client's problems and as a reminder to health care providers of things that need attention at each client contact. It also demonstrates the degree of sophistication of the practitioner's clinical judgment.

INITIAL PLANS

Delineating the initial plans for each problem forms the next logical step in the PORS. Each problem should have its own initial plan, titled and numbered according to the problem list, so that the experienced observer can quickly determine whether the problem has a complete and reasonable plan. Usually, the plan of action for a particular problem calls for additional diagnostic tests, specific therapeutic modalities, and the education of the client and the client's family. Or the plan may be simply to remain aware of the problem or to continue observing certain parameters of the problem.

PROGRESS NOTES

As the final component of the PORS, progress notes may appear in three ways: flow sheets, narrative notes, and discharge summaries. The acronym SOAP (subjective data, objective data, assessment, plan) was coined by a British physician, who reportedly said: "In England we're SOAPing the records—it helps to clean up the thinking, you see."[64] The SOAP format is always used in narrative notes and discharge summaries; flow sheets, however, may or may not use a SOAP format.

The goal of SOAPing is, indeed, to clarify thinking, to make apparent the rationale so that health professionals give better care to their clients. A major difference between progress notes in the PORS and traditional source-oriented narrative notes is the inclusion of the rationale. Seeing the logic or rationale behind the order for a specific medication, diagnostic exam, or laboratory test makes it more interesting and challenging for nurses to plan effective client-centered nursing care.

The subjective data of SOAP encompass all symptomatic data, or what the client or his or her family say, feel, or report. By placing the subjective data first, we make sure that the client's viewpoint gets considered from the beginning, for physicians tend to overlook the client and concentrate more on the ultrasound report or the lab finding.

The objective data result from your observations of the client, the physical examination, and the outcomes of diagnostic and laboratory studies. In effect, they are the tests, measurements, and physical signs that impress the practitioner's senses.

Flow sheets are valuable in recording and analyzing objective data in a graphic or tabular manner (Exhibit 2.18). They can be used whenever certain routine data or parameters of a problem will have recurrent observations (vital signs, fluid balance, electrolyte or oxygenation status).

When a client's condition is changing rapidly, a flow sheet may be the only progress note used. Some flow sheets can be prepared in advance for frequently seen problems such as diabetes, congestive heart failure, or myocardial infarction. Such highly structured flow charts provide an algorithm (or a set of procedural parameters) for the collection of data pertaining to specific problems. At other times, general-purpose flow sheets can be used whenever the health care providers desire to monitor the parameters that reflect the client's needs and physiological status.[65] As a

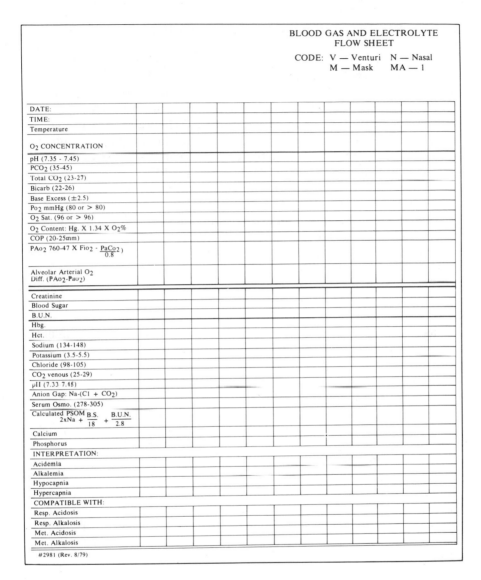

BLOOD GAS AND ELECTROLYTE
FLOW SHEET

CODE: V — Venturi   N — Nasal
M — Mask   MA — 1

DATE:											
TIME:											
Temperature											
O_2 CONCENTRATION											
pH (7.35 - 7.45)											
PCO_2 (35-45)											
Total CO_2 (23-27)											
Bicarb (22-26)											
Base Excess (±2.5)											
Po_2 mmHg (80 or > 80)											
O_2 Sat. (96 or > 96)											
O_2 Content: Hg. X 1.34 X $O_2\%$											
COP (20-25mm)											
PAo_2 760-47 X Fio_2 - $\frac{PaCo_2}{0.8}$)											
Alveolar Arterial O_2 Diff. $(PAo_2$-$Pao_2)$											
Creatinine											
Blood Sugar											
B.U.N.											
Hbg.											
Hct.											
Sodium (134-148)											
Potassium (3.5-5.5)											
Chloride (98-105)											
CO_2 venous (25-29)											
pH (7.33 7.45)											
Anion Gap: Na-(Cl + CO_2)											
Serum Osmo. (278-305)											
Calculated PSOM $2xNa + \frac{B.S.}{18} + \frac{B.U.N.}{2.8}$											
Calcium											
Phosphorus											
INTERPRETATION:											
Acidemia											
Alkalemia											
Hypocapnia											
Hypercapnia											
COMPATIBLE WITH:											
Resp. Acidosis											
Resp. Alkalosis											
Met. Acidosis											
Met. Alkalosis											

#2981 (Rev. 8/79)

Exhibit 2.18. Flow chart.

sufficient amount of data is collected on the flow sheet and analyzed in relation to the client's problem, the practitioner should write a periodic summary of it on the progress notes.[66]

The assessment portion of SOAP is your analysis or interpretation of the subjective and objective data. Because assessment demands a high level of cognitive skill—the ability to analyze, synthesize, and correlate causative factors, for example—it is not surprising that it is often difficult to do. Perhaps much of the difficulty stems from the fact that nurses are more accustomed to communicating assessments orally than to writing them down.[67] Above all, the most important point to remember here is that assessments have to be "logical and honest."[68] When various interpretations are really feasible on the PORS, go ahead and state them.

The plan portion of SOAP usually refers to the immediate plans related to the problem. It is the end product of logical thought about the subjective data, objective data, and assessment. Your plan might be to continue the original plan that the practitioner previously recorded to deal with the problem, or it might be to continue that modification of the original plan developed 2 days ago. Perhaps your plan will be to call for immediate help or for a consultation. As with the initial plans, the plan portion of SOAP can include further diagnostic studies, specific therapeutic actions, and client-family education.

In sum, the PORS orients all data around specific problems that alter health. As a logical and efficient way to organize and maintain data gathered for each client, it supplies a common bond among all health care providers involved in the client's care by allowing them to *communicate* through a made-to-order, logically organized system. The PORS begins with the compilation of the data base. This leads to the formulation of the problem list, which in turn generates the initial plans. The system incorporates a feedback loop from the progress notes to the problem list, to indicate the current status of a problem. If the progress notes show that problems #1 and #2 on the problem list are actually part of #5, this will be reflected on the revised problem list. The progress notes also produce a *feedback loop* to the initial plans. As practitioners "SOAP," they determine whether the initial plans require change or modification and they document the rationale for any modification. Ultimately, the methodology of logically analyzing problems in a SOAP format leads to another feedback loop between the progress notes and the data base. As new problems are identified in the progress notes, information previously gathered in the data base may be effectively used in the problem-solving process.

Guidelines for Writing PORS Progress Notes

We suggest seven guidelines for writing good PORS progress notes:

Guideline 1
Sign, date, and time all entries.

Guideline 2
Title each entry with a specific problem and/or number.

Guideline 3

Document transient episodes (which may or may not turn out to be new problems) under the heading "Temporary Problem" (Exhibit 2.19). Examples could be "leg cramps," "missing hearing aid," or "frontal headache."

			THE BARBERTON CITIZENS HOSPITAL NURSING PROGRESS RECORD
DATE	TIME	DATA	PERTINENT INFORMATION
11/10/81	1 PM	#5 Hypertension, secondary to CHF	
			S — None
			O — Admitting BP ® arm 190/90. During past 4 days BP has varied little from 110/70 – 120/70 (lying) to 116/70 – 110/84 (standing).
			A — Drug therapy is effective, c̄ minimal to no postural hypotension. Hypertension well controlled — possibly on low side for Mrs. J.?
			P — Ask physician regarding possibility of decreasing medication from BID to QD. J. Kraft, RN
11/10/81	6³⁰ Pm	Temporary Problem: Headache	
			S — "Bad headache over my eyes and in my neck."
			O — ² eyes tightly closed. BP ® arm 116/84 — sitting. Ate only half of supper. Family [treating] L.M. visited earlier.; told of plans to leave on vacation next week.
			A — Possible tension headache; possibly upset at family's plans to leave for vacation.
			P — ① Give prn med for headache. ② Close blinds. ③ Offer cold cloth or ice bag. ④ Recheck BP in 30 min. ⑤ Spend time with Mrs. J. before HS to talk about how she feels about vacation plans. L. Morris, RN

1094 (11-77)

Exhibit 2.19. Nursing progress entry (PORS style).

Guideline 4
Include all four elements in SOAP in your progress notes. If you are unable to get subjective data from the client, document the reason:

S—unresponsive

S—comatose

S—none

Guideline 5
Review flow sheet data at appropriate intervals and write a summary progress note.

Guideline 6
Include all pertinent sources of objective data when writing your progress notes, such as

- Vital signs
- Lab data
- Results of x-rays and noninvasive studies
- Physical findings, including results of inspection, palpation, percussion, and auscultation
- Psychological/emotional status—crying, affect, mood
- Signs—chills, diaphoresis; amount, color, and consistency of drainage from urinary catheters, chest tubes, wound drainage systems, and intermittent nasogastric suction
- Nonverbal communication modalities—eye contact, gestures, posture, dress

Guideline 7
Write progress notes whenever

- The client's condition changes
- The care plan or teaching plan is changed
- You observe anything unexpected
- An abnormality occurs, such as a dangerous cardiac arrhythmia, a high blood pressure reading, or an unusually low urinary output

DISCHARGE SUMMARIES

The nursing discharge summary serves two purposes. First, as an overview of the client's status upon discharge from the health care facility, it promotes the continuity of care and serves as a nursing referral to other professionals as they assume responsibility for the client's care. Second, it functions as a preliminary nursing audit since the nurse reviews the clinical record to summarize and evaluate the care that the client has received.

Discharge summaries may be written in either the problem-oriented format (Exhibit 2.20) or the narrative format (Exhibit 2.21). Some institutions, however, use printed semistructured forms to facilitate the documentation process (Exhibit 2.22). If the form does not supply enough space for all the client's problems, however, make a notation on it to refer others to the additional entry on the progress notes.

Keep in mind that the discharge summary briefly highlights the course of the client's progress throughout his or her contact with the agency. However, those problems that were never completely resolved should be documented more fully than those that responded favorably to nursing and medical interventions.

Consider the example of Mr. T. E., a 73-year-old retired farmer who was seen on four separate occasions in the outpatient clinic during the past year for management of several problems: hypertension, diabetes mellitus, an upper respiratory infection, and severe aching pain in his right leg. When Mr. T. E. decided to move to Florida to be near his son, he asked that his health record be forwarded to the new clinic he would be contacting. Gloria Murcia, his nurse, was asked to prepare his discharge summary. Since the hypertension and diabetes were under control and had not caused any untoward nursing or medical management problems, Gloria was able to document them easily.

On the other hand, the severe pain in Mr. T. E.'s right leg had consistently eluded management. Thus, Gloria and the internist with whom she worked summarized carefully the course of the problem, including the diagnostic measures taken to determine the etiology of the pain and the therapeutic measures to relieve it. Gloria also summarized nursing measures that had been somewhat successful in relieving the discomfort as well as those that had not helped at all. Consequently, their discharge summary about Mr. T. E.'s right leg pain was more involved and complete than that of his chronic (but successfully managed) problems so that the nurse and physician who would care for him in the future would have as much help as possible in knowing what nursing and medical interventions had been previously tried.

Whether you use the problem-oriented format or the narrative format, these five guidelines will help you write a discharge summary:

1. Before writing, review the client's progress throughout his or her hospitalization or contact with the agency.
2. Record the summary chronologically, beginning with the admission

DATE	TIME	DATA	PERTINENT INFORMATION
9/18/81		Discharge Summary:	
			S: Admitted 9/9/81 c̄ generalized lower abdominal pain which had become progressively worse during past 3 wks. To OR on 9/11/81 for D&C, Laparoscopy, and Ⓛ Salpingo-oophorectomy. Usual incisional discomfort now, but stated, "That awful pain is finally gone."
			O: Incision clean, dry, slightly edematous. No redness. Temperature 101.2° 24 hrs. post-op, but down to 98.8° 48 hrs. post-op (see flow-sheet). Has been ambulating in hall TID for past 72 hrs. c̄ help. For past 48 hrs. has received Empirin #3 tabs II c̄ good pain control. Constipated on 9/16. Enema given c̄ fair results.
			A: Wound healing. Edema at suture line within normal limits. Temporary constipation related to decreased activity and use of prns for pain.
			P: To go home for 4-5 weeks before returning to work. Mother will come for 1 wk. to help c̄ 5 yr. old son. Pt. ed.: Verbalized understanding of instructions to increase fiber in diet and to drink 8-10 glasses H₂O daily while taking Empirin. Rx for Empirin #3 and Colace 100 mg. given, along c̄ medication instruction sheet. Post-op gynecological discharge instruction sheet given and reviewed. Mrs. A. L. and husband verbalized their understanding of the instructions. ———— S. Miller, RN

1094 (11-77)

Exhibit 2.20. Discharge summary (problem-oriented format).

DATE	TIME	DATA	PERTINENT INFORMATION
9/18/81			Discharge Summary: Admitted 9/9/81 c̄ generalized lower abdominal pain. To OR on 9/11 for Ⓛ Salpingo-oophorectomy. Temp. was 101.2° on 9/12, but down to 98.8° by 9/13. Afebrile since. Other post-op vitals stable (see graphic flow sheet). Has been ambulating in hall for past 3 days s̄ assistance. Wound clean and dry; suture line slightly edematous. Incisional pain now controlled by Empirin #3 tabs ii q 4 hrs prn. Required enema on 9/16. Constipation related to decreased activity and effect of codeine on bowel motility. Instructed to drink 8-10 glasses of liquid daily and to increase fiber intake while on Empirin #3. Rx for Empirin #3 and Colace 100 mg. given, along c̄ medication instruction sheets. Instruction sheet for post-op gynecological surgeries given: To avoid stairs for 2-3 weeks; no heavy cleaning or lifting (such as laundry) for 3 weeks; no sexual activity for 6 weeks. May shower. No drug over incision. Both Ms. A.L. and husband verbalized knowledge of instructions and the signs and symptoms to report to the physician — fever, wound drainage, or swelling. To call today for appointment to see surgeon in 2 weeks. ——————— S. Miller, RN

1094 (11-77)

Exhibit 2.21. Discharge summary (narrative format).

DATE: 9/18/81   DISCHARGE   Home ☐   TIME OF DEATH_____
                 PLACEMENT: Nursing Home ☐
TIME: 9:30 Am   Other_____   Post Mortem: Yes ☐ No ☐
MODE: Ambulatory ☐   Person who came for patient Husband
       Wheelchair ☒   Transporter ☐
       Stretcher ☐   _____   Nursing Personnel ☐
                                                     Other_____

PATIENT CONDITION (Health Status): Check appropriate boxes:
Afebrile   ☒   Hygiene: Self Care ☒   Skin in Good Condition ☒
Free of Pain   ☐   Assist   ☐   Eating Well   ☐
Oriented (3 Spheres)   ☒   Total Care ☐   Taking Fluids Well   ☒
Appropriate Behavior   ☒   Able to Void   ☒
Ability to Function Independently ☒   Normal Defecation   ☐

Other: Appetite down, but has increased over past 48 hrs. Constipation (9/16)
related to decreased activity and oral pain medication.
Comments: Continues to have mild to moderate post-op incisional pain;
has been controlled by Empirin #3, tabs II.
Reaction to Discharge: "I'm glad to be going home."
Written Discharge - Yes ☒ No ☐
PATIENT ACTIVITY: Type and Extent of Activity: To avoid stairs for 2-3
Ambulatory   ☒   weeks. No heavy cleaning — no lifting of
Cane   ☐   laundry, babies over 15#, groceries.
Crutches   ☐   No driving for 4 weeks. No sexual
Walker   ☐   activity for 6 weeks.
Assistance   ☐   Understands Activity/Exercise:
Wheelchair   ☐   Patient: Yes ☒ No ☐ Family: Yes ☒ No ☐
Confined to Bed ☐
DIET: (↑ Fiber)   ADDITIONAL INFORMATION: Verbalized that she needs to
Name of Diet: General   increase fiber in diet (whole wheat bread,
Seen by Dietician: Yes ☐ fruits, vegetables) to prevent constipation.
                    No ☐
Understands Diet: Patient: Yes ☒ No ☐ Family: Yes ☒ No ☐
SPECIALIZED CARE - TREATMENTS: Type of Care and Instruction: Verbalized understanding
of the following: may shower; no drsg. over incision;
to call physician if suture line becomes edematous or
reddened or if it drains; or if she develops fever over
101° F. Post-op gynecological instruction sheet given to
A.L. and discussed with her and her family.

Understands Care: Patient: Yes ☒ No ☐ Family: Yes ☒ No ☐
Ability to perform: Patient: Yes ☒ No ☐ Family: Yes ☐ No ☐

Form 2751 (2/76)

Exhibit 2.22. Discharge summary, semistructured format (front).

MEDICATIONS:
(List)   (Instructions given to Patient/Family per each Drug)

Empirin #3 Ī or ĪĪ   Eat high fiber diet ; drink
q̄ 4 hrs. prn pain   8-10 glasses water daily since
                                      codeine can contribute to
                                      decreased bowel motility.

Colace 100 mg. po daily   Swallow tablet whole ; do not
as needed.   chew or crush it. Take the
                                      medicine at HS or in the early
                                      morning as it takes 6-10 hrs.
                                      to act.

Understands Medications: Patient: Yes ☒   No ☐   Family: Yes ☐   No ☐
Prescriptions Given: Yes ☒   No ☐   Filled at Hospital: Yes ☐   No ☐
Pre-Admission Drugs Returned: Yes ☐   No ☐   None ☒

REFERRAL:
Referral Made: Yes ☐   No ☒   Nursing Transfer Form Completed and sent: Yes ☐   No ☐
Type: _____

FOLLOW UP CARE.   Check appropriate box
Clinic Appointment ☐   Out-Patient Treatment ☐   M.D. Office Visit ☒
COMPLICATIONS ACQUIRED DURING HOSPITALIZATION: (List)
_____
_____
_____

                                      S. Miller   R.N.

IF PATIENT EXPIRES:

Family/Friend Notified   Yes ☐   Unable To Reach ☐   Minister/Priest Notified   Yes ☐   No ☐
Family/Friend Came   Yes ☐   No ☐

List of Valuables:
Glasses _____   Luggage _____
Teeth _____   Watch _____
Money _____   Wallet _____   (R.N.)
Rings _____   Keys _____   Personal Belongings were given to:
Clothing_____   Others: _____

Exhibit 2.22. Discharge summary, semistructured format (back).

(or first contact with the agency), and systematically highlight the client's progress.

3. Refer other professionals to flow sheets or graphic records for unusual details or occurrences.

4. Write a separate narrative or problem-oriented entry for each problem. For instance, the client who has a fractured right tibia and a urinary tract infection should have a separate discharge summary for each of the problems.

5. Document your discharge teaching activities and your client's and/or family's understanding of self-care activities or instructions.

SUMMARY

Effective client-centered documentation is based on the four phases of the nursing process: assessment, planning, implementation, and evaluation.

Nursing assessments incorporate the collection and recording of subjective (history-taking) data as well as objective (observational) data to serve as a framework for formulating clients' health care management. Well-designed assessment tools help the professional nurse collect and document information efficiently.

As the end product of the assessment phase of the nursing process, a nursing diagnosis is a clear, concise statement describing the client's actual or potential health problem that nurses, by virtue of their educational preparation and licensure, are capable of treating. A nursing diagnosis may be stated in terms of the problem, its cause or etiology, and its associated signs and symptoms.

Care plans are the written results of the planning stage of the nursing process. Care plans relate the nursing diagnosis or problem, long- and short-term goals to resolve the problem, and specific interventions or nursing orders to treat the problem and achieve the goals. An evaluation column is often added to the care plan to ensure that all four phases of the nursing process are used in planning client-centered care.

As the primary communication tool at the nurse's disposal, written care plans provide for consistent, ordered, and continuous care. They must be updated regularly for clients and nurses to receive full benefit from the tool.

Client-centered goals are often referred to as expected outcomes. Nurses write long-term goals as criteria to predict the client's behavior during the restorative phase of illness. Derived from long-term goals, short-term goals predict in a measurable, quantifiable way the client's behavior by a certain target date.

Well-written nursing orders give direction to the implementation of the nursing care plan. Initiated with an action verb, they must answer questions of specificity—*who, when, what, how much,* and *how long.*

Teaching plans represent another facet of the planning phase of the nursing process. Succinctly written teaching guides help the nurse plan more effective teaching-learning situations and be better prepared for spontaneous teaching opportunities.

Nurses write standard teaching plans in many agencies to unify the basic instructional content. Yet because clients have unique learning needs that cannot be predicted until they are individually assessed, nurses must also know how to modify standard teaching plans and write individual plans. A three-column format can serve as a viable tool in writing meaningful teaching plans.

As an integral part of teaching plans, clearly written performance objectives are stated in terms of what the learner must be able to do, perform, or achieve to attain the learning goal. Performance objectives specify not only the conditions under which the behavior is to be achieved but also the criteria or standards against which the performance can be measured or evaluated. Verbs open to few interpretations in meaning help the nurse write clear, concise objectives.

The documentation process provides the written record of the implementation and the evaluation phases of the nursing process. The source-oriented (narrative) system and the problem-oriented system are the two types of documentation formats currently in use.

In the source-oriented system, notes are written in a narrative style, following a strict chronological order. In the problem-oriented system, entries are made according to identified client problems. The acronym SOAP forms the basis for recording subjective and objective data, the assessment or analysis of the data, and the plan of care on the progress record. Well-designed flow sheets may be used with either system to facilitate the collection, recording, and analysis of data related to specific aspects of client care.

Discharge summaries constitute one aspect of the fourth phase of the nursing process, evaluation. Written in either the problem-oriented or narrative format, they summarize the progress and nursing care the client has received throughout his or her contact with the health care facility. Semistructured discharge assessment forms can also ease the nurse's role in effective documentation.

EXERCISES

1. Using either your agency's admission assessment tool or the one given in Exhibit 2.2, write an admission assessment for a client you have cared for recently. Evaluate the effectiveness of your assessment by asking other professionals to read it and critique it.
2. Write a meaningful nursing diagnosis for a client you have cared for recently, based on one of the following accepted diagnostic categories:
   - Alterations in comfort
   - Impairment of digestion
   - Fear
   - Fluid volume deficit
   - Impaired thought processes

   Use Gordon's PES format to state the client's actual or potential health problem, the etiology, and the signs and symptoms. Recall that accepted diagnostic categories are broad in scope and that you will probably need to individualize the diagnosis to make it meaningful to the client you have cared for.

3. Analyze and critique a standard teaching plan from your health care facility that has been developed for a selected group of clients—for example, newly diagnosed hypertensives, those with chronic obstructive lung disease, or those undergoing elective surgery. Then revise the plan or develop your own according to the guidelines given in the text. Consider how you would adapt the plan to meet specific individual needs as well as to fit the needs of a diverse group of clients.

4. Each of the following statements describes a teaching technique. Rewrite them to reflect specific learner-centered performance objectives, including the criteria for each one. Whenever appropriate, include the conditions for attaining each objective.

   a. Teach the mother how to take a radial pulse and check to be sure that she gets the same results as the nurse.
   b. Instruct the client in the mechanics of crutch walking.
   c. Inform the learner about foods high in potassium.
   d. Teach Mr. J. three signs of pacemaker failure, as listed in the pamphlet "All About Your Pacemaker."
   e. Show the family how to change a Foley catheter.
   f. Develop in the husband the ability to give his wife tube feedings.
   g. Demonstrate quadriceps-setting exercises to the client, which he is to do every hour during the day.
   h. Encourage the client to express her fears about surgery.

5. Ms. K. T., a 50-year-old client with severe degenerative joint disease, had a total joint arthroplasty of her left hip. Given the nursing diagnosis of "impaired mobility of both legs and buttocks related to use of postoperative abduction pillow," complete Ms. T.'s care plan. Include one long-term goal, two or three short-term goals, and at least four nursing orders to implement the care plan.

6. Critique, analyze, and rewrite when necessary the following nursing orders:

   a. Encourage fluids.
   b. Spend time daily with client.
   c. Listen for bowel sounds.
   d. Take BP in (L) arm each shift.
   e. Teach client about medications.
   f. Have Ms. J. do her exercises × 2.
   g. Give emotional support as needed.
   h. Reward Mrs. K. whenever she chooses the right foods.

7. Critique the following entries from selected care plans and revise them according to the principles of formulating nursing diagnoses or problems, short-term goals, and nursing orders.

a. 1/5	Inadequate information about post D & C bleeding.	Will understand information presented about duration of post D & C flow.	1. Tell pt. the usual duration of post D & C flow. 2. Teach pt. to recognize abnormal postop flow.
b. 3/21	Cannot talk because of stroke.	Teach client to communicate by discharge date.	1. Let pt. write notes if possible. 2. Let her point to pictures of items on felt board.
c. 7/18	Discomfort (L) ear related to tinnitus.	Discomfort will decrease.	1. Position on unaffected side. 2. Check ears c̄ otoscope.

8. Critique the following narrative notes and rewrite them as necessary to reflect more meaningful communication.

a. 4/12/80   9:30 AM   Refused medication. Stated it made her sick.

   10:00 AM   Ambulated in hall—didn't do as well as yesterday.

   10:30 AM   Had large emesis.

   12:30 PM   Refused lunch. Stated she felt nauseated.

   2:30 PM   Better. Fair day.

b. 9/26/80   8:00 PM   Vital signs good. Moving legs, but c/o numbness.

   9:00 PM   Voided lge. amt. straw-colored urine. C/o pain, but refuses med.

   10:00 PM   Still c/o pain, but refusing shot. Very uncomfortable.

   2/27/80   12:30 AM   Seems to be sleeping.

9. Write a problem-oriented entry for each of the following nursing diagnoses or problems:

   a. Impaired sleep pattern related to lumbosacral pain

   b. Moderate anxiety related to fear of impending surgery

c. Impaired verbal communication related to edema of larynx

d. Inadequate information related to drug allergy

e. Potential gastric irritation related to large doses of aspirin therapy

10. Write both a problem-oriented and a source-oriented discharge summary for Mr. T. E., the 73-year-old retired farmer. Details of his problems are given in the text in the section on discharge summaries.

REFERENCES

1. Dolores E. Little and Doris L. Carnevali, *Nursing Care Planning,* 2d ed. (Philadelphia: Lippincott, 1976), p. 230.

2. Maria C. Phaneuf, *The Nursing Audit: Profile for Excellence* (New York: Appleton-Century-Crofts, 1972), pp. 15–18.

3. Little and Carnevali, p. 122.

4. Ann Marriner, *The Nursing Process: A Scientific Approach To Nursing Care,* 2d ed. (St. Louis: Mosby, 1979), pp. 31–32.

5. Little and Carnevali, pp. 124–125.

6. Derry A. Moritz, "Nursing Histories—A Guide, Yes. A Form, No!" *Oncology Nursing Forum,* 6 (Fall 1979), 18.

7. Noella Devolder McCray, "Assessment Tools: Oncology Patient Assessment Tool," *Oncology Nursing Forum,* 6 (Fall 1979), 15.

8. Mary Blount and others, "Documenting With the Problem-oriented Record System," *American Journal of Nursing,* 78 (September 1978), 1540.

9. Little and Carnevali, pp. 141–142.

10. Little and Carnevali, p. 105.

11. Little and Carnevali, p. 141.

12. Ellen Thomas Eggland, "How to Take a Meaningful Nursing History," *Nursing77,* 7 (July 1977), 27.

13. Marjory Gordon, "Nursing Diagnoses and the Diagnostic Process," *American Journal of Nursing,* 76 (August 1976), 1298.

14. Mary Radatovich Price, "Nursing Diagnosis: Making a Concept Come Alive," *American Journal of Nursing,* 80 (April 1980), 668.

15. Gordon, p. 1298.

16. Price, p. 669.

17. Gordon, p. 1298.

18. Gordon, p. 1298.

19. Mary O'Neil Mundinger and Grace Dotterer Jauron, "Developing a Nursing Diagnosis," *Nursing Outlook,* 23 (February 1975), 96.

20. Mundinger and Jauron, p. 97.

21. Rudy L. Ciuca, "Over the Years With the Nursing Care Plan," *Nursing Outlook,* 20 (November 1972), 706.
22. Little and Carnevali, p. 268.
23. Marlene G. Mayers, *A Systematic Approach to the Nursing Care Plan,* 2d ed. (New York: Appleton-Century-Crofts, 1978), p. 26.
24. June T. Bailey and Karen E. Claus, *Decision Making in Nursing: Tools for Change* (St. Louis: Mosby, 1975), p. 34.
25. Price, p. 671.
26. Mayers, pp. 33–36.
27. Philip C. Kolin and Janeen L. Kolin, *Professional Writing for Nurses in Education, Practice, and Research* (St. Louis: Mosby, 1980), p. 39.
28. Grace L. Deloughery, *History and Trends of Professional Nursing,* 8th ed. (St. Louis: Mosby, 1977), p. 58.
29. Stanley G. Rosenberg, "Patient Education: An Educator's View," in *Compliance With Therapeutic Regimens,* eds. David L. Sackett and R. Brian Haynes (Baltimore: Johns Hopkins University Press, 1976), p. 93.
30. Minnie Goodnow, *The Technic of Nursing,* 3d ed. (Philadelphia: Saunders, 1935), p. 58.
31. Goodnow, p. 61.
32. Barbara Klug Redman, *The Process of Patient Teaching in Nursing,* 3d ed. (St. Louis: Mosby, 1976), pp. 1–2.
33. G. Maureen Chaisson, "Patient Education: Whose Responsibility Is It and Who Should Be Doing It?" *Nursing Administration Quarterly,* 4 (Winter 1980), 1–2.
34. Tamar Gilson-Parkevich, "Focus on Patient Education," in *Patient and Family Education: Tools, Techniques, and Theory,* eds. Rose-Marie Duda McCormick and Tamar Gilson-Parkevich (New York: Wiley, 1979), pp. 5–10.
35. Laurel Ratcliff Talabere, "The Challenge of Patient and Family Teaching," in *Patient and Family Education: Tools, Techniques, and Theory,* eds. Rose-Marie Duda McCormick and Tamar Gilson-Parkevich (New York: Wiley, 1979), p. 19.
36. Margaret L. Pohl, *The Teaching Function of the Nursing Practitioner,* 3d ed. (Dubuque, IA: Brown, 1978), p. 127.
37. Chaisson, p. 3.
38. See Karen S. Zander and others, *Practical Manual for Patient-Teaching* (St. Louis: Mosby, 1978), for many examples of standard teaching plans.
39. Redman, p. 163.
40. Pohl, pp. 53–54.
41. Lilah Harper, "Developing and Evaluating a Patient Education Program," in *Patient Education* (New York: National League for Nursing, 1976), p. 4.
42. Robert F. Mager, *Preparing Instructional Objectives,* 2d ed. (Belmont, CA: Fearon, 1975), p. 24.
43. John P. De Cecco and William R. Crawford, *The Psychology of Learning and*

Instruction: Educational Psychology, 2d ed. (Englewood Cliffs, NJ: Prentice-Hall, 1974), p. 28.

44. Doris Nuttelman, "Instructional Objectives," *Supervisor Nurse,* 8 (November 1977), 35.
45. Redman, pp. 69–78.
46. Mager, pp. 43–45.
47. Mager, p. 21.
48. Goodnow, pp. 168–169.
49. Goodnow, p. 170.
50. Aline MacDonnell Holmes, "Problem-oriented Medical Records, Nursing Audit and Accountability," *Supervisor Nurse,* 11 (April 1980), 40.
51. Delores Thoma and Karen Pittman, "Evaluation of Problem-oriented Nursing Notes," *Journal of Nursing Administration,* 2 (May–June 1972), 50.
52. Mary D. Hemelt and Mary Ellen Mackert, "Factual Medical Records Protect Hospitals, Practitioners, Patients," *Hospitals,* 51 (July 1, 1977), 50.
53. Hemelt and Mackert, p. 52.
54. F. R. Woolley and others, *Problem-oriented Nursing* (New York: Springer, 1974), p. 4.
55. Judith T. Bloom and others, "Problem-oriented Charting," *American Journal of Nursing,* 71 (November 1971), 2145.
56. Holmes, p. 42.
57. Margaret Ireland, "Meaningful Nurses Notes," *Nursing Homes,* 23 (February–March 1974), 16.
58. Marilyn T. Hansen, "Make Your Charting the 'Topic-of-the-Day,' " *Nursing76,* 6 (May 1976), 74.
59. Lawrence L. Weed, *Medical Records, Medical Education, and Patient Care: The Problem-oriented Record as a Basic Tool* (Cleveland: Case Western Reserve University, 1969), pp. 4–6.
60. Weed, p. 6.
61. Jacques L. Sherman, Jr., and Sylvia Kleiman Fields, *Guide to Patient Evaluation: History Taking, Physical Examination, and the Problem-oriented Method,* 3d ed. (Garden City, NY: Medical Examination Publishing, 1978), p. 17.
62. Weed, p. 27.
63. Stephen R. Yarnall and Judith Atwood, "Problem-oriented Practice for Nurses and Physicians: General Concepts," *Nursing Clinics of North America,* 9 (June 1974), 220.
64. Mary Woody and Mary Mallison, "The Problem-oriented System for Patient-centered Care," *American Journal of Nursing,* 73 (July 1973), 1172.
65. Mary Blount and others, "Documenting With the Problem-oriented Record System," *American Journal of Nursing,* 78 (September 1978), 1542. See also Maureen B. Niland and Patricia M. Bentz, "A Problem-oriented Approach to Planning Nursing Care," *Nursing Clinics of North America,* 9 (June 1974), 238.
66. Timothy Porter O'Grady, "Problem Oriented Charting: The Educational and Implementation Challenge," *Supervisor Nurse,* 8 (January 1977), 18.

67. Woody, p. 1173.
68. Holmes, p. 43.

FURTHER READING

Ansley, Betty. "Patient-oriented Recording: A Better System for Ambulatory Settings." *Nursing75,* 5 (August 1975), 52–53.

Bartos, Louise T., and Marie Ray Knight. "Documentation of Nursing Process." *Supervisor Nurse,* 9 (July 1978), 41–48.

Bloom, Benjamin S., ed. *Taxonomy of Educational Objectives: The Classification of Educational Goals. Handbook I: Cognitive Domain.* New York: McKay, 1956.

Campbell, Claire. *Nursing Diagnosis and Intervention in Nursing Practice.* New York: Wiley, 1978.

Creighton, Helen. "Nurse's Charting—Part I." *Supervisor Nurse,* 11 (May 1980), 42–43.

———. "Nurse's Charting—Part II." *Supervisor Nurse,* 11 (June 1980), 61–62.

Fouts, Joan. "The Teaching Square." *Supervisor Nurse,* 9 (December 1978), 12–13.

Gordon, Marjory, Mary Anne Sweeney, and Kathleen McKeehan. "Nursing Diagnosis: Looking at Its Use in the Clinical Area." *American Journal of Nursing,* 80 (April 1980), 672–674.

Hamilton, Ann, and Patricia Kelley. "An Educational Program for Hysterectomy Patients." *Supervisor Nurse,* 10 (April 1979), 19–21, 25.

Henderson, Virginia. "On Nursing Care Plans and Their History." *Nursing Outlook,* 21 (June 1973), 378–379.

Mancini, Marguerite. "Documenting Clinical Records." *American Journal of Nursing,* 78 (September 1978), 1556, 1561.

Reilly, Dorothy E. *Behavioral Objectives in Nursing: Evaluation of Learner Attainment.* New York: Appleton-Century-Crofts, 1975.

Schell, Pamela L., and Alla T. Campbell. "POMR—Not Just Another Way to Chart." *Nursing Outlook,* 20 (August 1972), 510–514.

Shuler, Cynthia. "Documenting Patient Teaching." *Supervisor Nurse,* 10 (June 1979), 43, 47–49.

Smith, Dorothy M. "Writing Objectives as a Nursing Practice Skill." *American Journal of Nursing,* 71 (February 1971), 319–320.

Tyzenhouse, Phyllis. "Care Plans for Nursing Home Patients." *Nursing Outlook,* 20 (March 1972), 169–172.

Whitehouse, Rebecca. "Forms That Facilitate Patient Teaching." *American Journal of Nursing,* 79 (July 1979), 1227–1229.

Zimmerman, Donna, and Carol Gohrke. "The Goal Directed Nursing Approach: It Does Work." *American Journal of Nursing,* 70 (February 1970), 306–310.

CHAPTER III

Writing Readable
Health Information
for the Client

Objectives

After studying this chapter, you will be able to

1. Discuss the interrelationship between audience analysis and written health education materials.
2. State four factors to consider in analyzing a selected audience.
3. Discuss five demographic variables that contribute to effective audience analysis.
4. Define the importance of readability as it applies to health education materials.
5. State factors that enhance and impair the readability of written health information.
6. Discuss the advantages and disadvantages of four commonly used readability formulas.
7. Apply the Gunning Fog Index, the SMOG formula, and the cloze procedure to selected reading samples.
8. Discuss the importance of selecting an appropriate format when writing client-centered health education materials.
9. Apply the 15 general guidelines for writing health education materials to evaluate the effectiveness of commercially prepared information.
10. Write an instructional and/or informational fact sheet based on principles of readability and audience analysis.
11. Write clear discharge instructions.
12. Discuss the guidelines for writing about medications.
13. Compose appropriate medication instructions for a selected audience.
14. State the components of a nurse-client contract.
15. Develop a nurse-client contract to use in your clinical practice.

Now more than ever, professional nurses are involved in selecting, using, evaluating, and even composing written health care information for their clients. A wide variety of written information is available on many health education topics and, as a nurse educator involved in client teaching, you need to know how to choose written information wisely to best meet the needs of your client population.

Written materials about specific problems or aspects of care can greatly aid the learning process. These materials remain available to clients after they leave the health care facility and so reinforce and supplement the teaching done by the health professional.[1] They provide a written reminder of the details of self-care instructions that clients often forget in the pressure of a "health crisis" situation.

It is essential for health care providers to realize that written information cannot supplant the teaching-learning activities that occur face to face between nurse educator and client. Written materials used alone do not provide the opportunity for the client to ask questions and, in turn, for the nurse to evaluate the client's understanding of the material. But as reinforcement for oral instructions or teaching sessions, written information can be extremely valuable.

Although many national organizations, such as the American Cancer Society and the American Heart Association, have developed quality materials for the general public on serious health problems, nurses at many agencies often cooperate in designing and writing client education materials to better meet the needs of their specific audience. In the late 1970s, nurses at the University Health Service, University of Wisconsin—Madison, developed health education materials on the common cold, mononucleosis, and strep throat, among others, specifically to fulfill the needs of the clinic's young adult population.[2] Because this population expects information about health maintenance and disease prevention, the details, content, and vocabulary used in this series of leaflets would not be appropriate for another client population, such as Hispanics in a large urban center.

To cite another situation, it is not surprising that the search in the late 1960s by *Nursing Outlook* author Jo-Ann Townsend for suitable educational literature for the pregnant adolescent proved almost futile. There was nothing available that met the specific needs of the unmarried expectant teenager. Furthermore, her survey showed that available prenatal literature was geared toward the middle-class suburban couple, not toward the urban couple at the lower end of the socioeconomic scale.[3] In her article, Townsend urges the development of appropriate and realistic literature for the unmarried pregnant adolescent.

In this chapter, then, we will focus on writing readable health information for the client. Topics we can profitably consider include audience analysis, readability formulas, format selection, general guidelines for writing health education materials, writing clear instructions and readable information, writing about medications, and writing nurse-client contracts.

AUDIENCE ANALYSIS

Successful writers in *all* fields never lose sight of the people for whom they are writing. They remain constantly aware of their target audience or selected population, whether it is composed of engineers, physicians, legal secretaries, or architects. Writers who have analyzed their audience and have taken into account its special problems, concerns, and needs, as well as its general reading level, do a more effective job of conveying their message. Such writers want their audience to comprehend the message, react to it, and possibly complete the communication loop by some specific action so that they know their intended message was understood.

In order to be successful when you write health education materials for your clients, you must have a clear idea of the audience you are trying to reach. Are you writing a pamphlet for the young teenager recently diagnosed as having scoliosis, or are you writing baby care instructions for the young mother? Ideally, you would approach writing a pamphlet on hypertension for young to middle-aged black males from a large inner-city tenement complex differently from writing one for senior citizens in an upper middle class retirement village. In fact, written materials supplementing health education activities become more effective as they are adapted to the needs of a specific audience or client population.

Even in highly specialized ambulatory outpatient facilities, however, it is obvious that *no* audience is completely homogeneous. If the facility serves a large number of arthritis clients, for instance, how does it determine what factors, besides arthritis, contribute to the make-up of its client population? What factors, in short, should you be aware of before devising written materials for your clients?

First, you should analyze the audience by surveying or sampling the demographic data from your facility's admitting records. Useful items to examine include

- *Age.* In addition to age, you can also consider average age and age span. And if your clients are children, you need to weigh carefully the developmental and maturational factors, too.
- *Ethnicity.* Your clients' cultural background can have a tremendous impact on their ability to read, speak, and understand English, for example.
- *Socioeconomic Status.* Your clients' social and economic background may greatly influence their willingness to enter the health care system and to learn how to manage self-care activities.
- *Educational Background.* There is a fairly predictable correlation between a person's educational background and his or her reading level.
- *Physiological Status.* Elderly diabetic clients will probably have some degree of visual impairment and so may not be able to read small print. Or perhaps clients with chronic obstructive pulmonary disease will not be able to absorb complexly written health information because of a decreased supply of oxygen to the brain.

These items can help you determine just how uniform your audience is. The greater the variation in client population, the more difficult it will be to write to one specific audience. However, certain guidelines will be discussed later that can help you write well to a somewhat heterogeneous audience.

The second factor to consider when writing health education materials for an audience is the purpose of your writing. Will you be writing medication instructions, home care instructions, or informational fact sheets? Knowing *why* you want to write helps you more realistically analyze your audience.

Learning needs make up the third factor to consider in writing appropriately for your client population. Here you seek to discover what your audience's experiences have been in relation to exposure to previous health teaching. Questions to ask yourself in analyzing informational or learning needs include the following:

- *What is the audience's existing knowledge base?* For instance, are there significant numbers of clients in your audience who have cared for or helped care for other diabetic family members? If so, what information and attitudes are they transferring from previous experience that will now influence their own health maintenance? The audience's existing knowledge base may be broad and accurate, may be nonexistent, or may contain many misconceptions.

- *What does the audience want to learn?* If the audience is composed chiefly of adults, it is crucial to find out what their concerns are and what they want to learn about a health problem. Adults will be more likely to read and learn what you have written if it addresses topics that the majority of the audience want to learn about. Over half of the parents surveyed by John W. Scanlon, as reported in his 1971 article for *Clinical Pediatrics,* indicated that the kind of information they would want to know, if they were told their child had an innocent heart murmur, revolved around diet and activity modification.[4] Thus, these concerns could be appropriately addressed both in teaching sessions with the child and parents and in written information. But until an audience is surveyed to find out what it would want to learn about a particular health problem, it is quite possible for health care providers to overlook its concerns.

- *What does the audience need to know?* Stressing what your clients need to know—as opposed to what it might be "nice" to know—will help keep you on target when you plan written information. A pamphlet that reinforces the nurse educator's teaching session with a newly diagnosed insulin-dependent diabetic *must* emphasize the possible symptoms of a hypoglycemic reaction and what measures to take if a reaction occurs. This is essential "survival" information for the recently diagnosed diabetic. Such persons need to know what to do and whom to call should they have a hypoglycemic reaction after leaving the hospital. What they do *not* need to know at this time, according to diabetes experts, is foot care technique.[5] The relationship between hygiene and complications is best taught during the home management phase of client education. So, for written information to be most effective, it must match the client's teaching-learning needs.

The fourth factor to consider in audience analysis is what Marjorie M. Crow and her co-authors call the "emotional components of human behavior." They maintain that it is not enough simply to present "information with precision, accuracy, logic, and clarity," for too often it fails to be read, to be remembered, or to effect behavioral change.[6]

In analyzing the client population attending the family planning program at Grady Memorial Hospital in Atlanta, Crow and her colleagues discovered that in terms of education, age, and number of children, the audience at the clinic matched the profile of women who read "confession" magazines. Furthermore, preliminary studies by these health educators revealed that women attending the family planning clinic did indeed read confession magazines on a regular basis. And so the educators developed a 30-page confession-format magazine called *True to Life*.

The central purpose of *True to Life* was to encourage women who already used contraceptives to continue to use them. To this end, stories stressing the emotional components of human behavior—loneliness, lack of communication, emotional dependency—appeared. The success of *True to Life* seems attributable to its emotional or human interest appeal to its intended audience, not to the factual information that the stories contained.[7]

Although few nurse educators might have the time or resources to devote to as big a project as the confession magazine developed at Grady Memorial, they should at least consider the emotional components of human behavior an important factor in promoting audience interest in and acceptance of written health information. It is possible, for example, that men who enjoy outdoor sports could benefit from a "sports page approach" to hypertensive health education information.

READABILITY FORMULAS

Once you have analyzed your audience, how do you make sure that you write health education materials so that your audience can understand them? Most authorities agree that the critical element to consider at this point is readability. Just how easy is it for the audience to read and understand the written information?

Importance of Readability

The authors of *An Overview of Adult Education Research* point out that Professors W. S. Gray and B. Leary did the first systematic research on the question of readability during the 1930s at the University of Chicago. In attempting to discover what it was in writing that caused difficulties in reading, Gray and Leary found just about what you might expect: (1) long intricate sentences and (2) unusual polysyllabic words.[8]

Readability first became more than an academic concept during World War II when large quantities of important information on the allied war effort needed to be communicated as clearly and as quickly as possible to average Americans. During that time, sentences in several of this country's newspapers were averaging well over 20 words long, making it difficult for readers to plow through the long columns. In fact, the readability of the average newspaper matched the complexity of *Atlantic Monthly* prose at an eleventh or twelfth grade reading level.[9] Although many readers *could* read and understand the messages, many others *did not feel like* making an effort to do so. Pioneers in developing and adapting readability formulas for newspapers, businesses, and law firms include Rudolf Flesch and Robert Gunning.

Among the solid reasons for being concerned about readability when preparing written health education materials, the most obvious is that clients who cannot understand instructions written at the fifth grade level will derive no benefit from your carefully prepared leaflet if it is written at the twelfth grade level. Furthermore, clients who normally have no difficulty reading and comprehending most materials at the twelfth grade level may have considerable difficulty if the crisis of their health problem has made it harder for them to comprehend what they normally would have no trouble with.

Readability studies conducted with selected client audiences have yielded some startling results. For instance, Mary Mohammed's classic 1964 study of 300 outpatients attending a diabetes clinic at University Hospitals of Cleveland shows that only 22% of this population could read and understand materials written at the eighth grade level.[10] Leonard and Cecilia Doak report in *The Diabetes Educator* that the "median literacy level of the U.S. population is approximately at the 10th grade." Even so, one-fifth of the adult population is functionally illiterate, that is, reads at the fifth grade level or lower.[11] Although several researchers agree that the number of years of schooling seems to be the "best prediction of reading ability,"[12] there is often a gap between the reading level and the years of schooling completed. The person who finished high school may read at the eighth grade level, for example.

What determines how "readable" a booklet or pamphlet is? We have already implied that short sentences (averaging 14–15 words) and familiar words make information more appealing, hence, more readable. But interest in a topic and the desire to know more about it also influence readability. The client who is highly motivated to learn all he can about diabetes is more likely to read the more difficult material than is the unmotivated client who is given only information written at, or just slightly below, his or her reading level. And if the material is far below the reader's level, the person will probably skim over large sections of it and miss essential information. Clearly, short sentences and familiar terms do not necessarily promote readability, especially if the overall effect is one of monotony. Most reading experts advocate varying sentence length and judiciously introducing and defining new terms to enliven the material.

Format also affects readability. Such potentially valuable items as headings, illustrations, charts, graphs, type size, color of print, and amount of white space on a page can increase the visual appeal and readability of prepared materials.

Stylistic factors may also contribute to increased or decreased readability. In *The Art of Readable Writing,* Rudolf Flesch shows how replacing "heavy" prepositions, conjunctions, and connectives with simpler, more easily understood words will greatly strengthen writing style and improve the case with which your audience reads and understands your prose.[13] For example, you can often use *so* instead of *accordingly, consequently, for this reason, hence,* and *thus.* And you can replace the longer or "heavier" terms *in favor of, in order to,* and *with a view to* with just *to.* The word *about* does the job more simply than *with regard to, with reference to,* and *in the neighborhood of.*

Researchers Richard R. Lanese and Randolph S. Thrush, as well as other reading experts in adult health education, repeatedly single out word difficulty and sentence length as the two biggest variables affecting readability.[14] As far as the first variable is concerned, we might say that unfamiliar words or terms are "difficult."

Now word difficulty has a special significance for health educators because our professional vocabulary contains many nursing and medical terms that both well-educated and less well-educated clients have difficulty in understanding. And so health writers often consult the "Dale List of 3,000 Familiar Words" when they write client-centered information. Robert Gunning reprints this list at the end of his book, *The Technique of Clear Writing.*[15] Prepared by Dr. Edgar Dale of Ohio State University, this list includes words familiar to at least 80% of the tested fourth grade students. While it may be impossible to write health materials choosing *only* from the "familiar" words, the Dale list at least supplies one guideline for assessing vocabulary difficulty. The list may also help a writer determine how to introduce and define unfamiliar medical or health terms so that they can be understood by the reader.

In light of our discussion so far, we believe that you would profit by reading Thrush and Lanese's "The Use of Printed Material in Diabetes Education," an article that appeared in *Diabetes* in 1962. After analyzing 143 samples of printed material designed to help diabetic clients understand their condition, the authors determined that approximately one word in every five was "unfamiliar to the diabetic with less than a fifth grade education—a majority of clinical or service patients."[16] From the Thrush-Lanese list (which starts with such words as *insulin, diabetes, diet,* and *urine*), you will see the variety and frequency of words that are "unfamiliar" to many diabetic clients.[17] Clearly, writers preparing diabetic education materials would want to review this word list.

Survey of Readability Formulas

Several readability formulas have been developed to help writers estimate the reading difficulty of written materials. Two early efforts, the Flesch Readability Formula and the Gunning Fog Index, rely heavily on sentence and word length to determine reading levels. But we must remember that any readability formula serves only as "a simple warning system." It cannot measure the quality of writing but only, to a limited extent, its complexity. As Robert Gunning so aptly states, "Nonsense written simply is still nonsense."[18] Readability formulas do not distinguish between precise terms and vague terms or between familiar words and less well-known words. They do measure word length, and the general assumption is that the longer the word, the more complex it is. If you view readability formulas as only guidelines to help you assess the complexity of your writing, they can prove useful in estimating the difficulty of your writing.

Developed in the early 1940s, the Flesch formula was originally based on three factors, namely, average sentence length, a count of references to people, and a count of prefixes and suffixes as an indicator of word difficulty. Yet the formula was flawed, for frequently two people making an analysis of the same sample would come up with a different number of prefixes and suffixes. Eventually, the formula required the counting of *all syllables*. But because of the tedious nature of having to check a dictionary to be sure that all syllables were correctly counted, the Flesch formula has often been criticized as too time-consuming. You can find out more about this rather involved formula by reading the appendix to *The Art of Readable Writing*.[19]

Later in the 1940s, Gunning developed the famous Fog Index when his consulting firm, Robert Gunning Associates, was set up to help publication staffs improve their writing. Gunning's formula is easy to use and is especially helpful in determining the readability of shorter pieces.

To determine the Fog Index of a passage, follow these three steps:

1. Use a passage of at least 100 words. If the piece is long, take several samples of 100 words each, spaced evenly throughout the writing, to give a more reliable score. Divide the number of words in a passage by the number of sentences, to give the average sentence length. Count independent clauses—separated by semicolons, dashes, or colons, but not commas—as separate sentences.

2. For each passage of about 100 words, count the number of three-syllable (or more) words. Don't count (1) capitalized words, (2) words that are combinations of short, easy words (such as *buttonhole, butterfly,* or *teenager*), and (3) verb forms made three syllables long by adding *ed* or *es* (such as *maintained* or *created*). Divide the number of three-syllable (or more) words—the so-called hard words—by the total number of words in the sample to get the percentage of hard words.

3. Add the average sentence length and the percentage of hard words, then multiply by .4. The resulting figure is the Fog Index, or readability score of a passage, expressed in reading grade level.[20]*

Early in *The Technique of Clear Writing,* Gunning compares several magazines and their grade levels as determined by the Fog Index. In the easy-reading range, he lists comics (sixth grade, or Fog Index of 6), *Ladies' Home Journal* (eighth grade, or Fog Index of 8), *Reader's Digest* (tenth grade, or Fog Index of 10), and *Time* (eleventh grade, junior in high school, or Fog Index of 11). Writing above the twelfth grade level, he maintains, exceeds the "danger line,"[21] for few people in the audience will be able to—or want to—take the time necessary to understand the message. As a point of reference, you should know that *Harper's* and *Atlantic Monthly* are written at the twelfth grade level but that no popular magazines are written above the high school senior level.

Unlike the Flesch and Gunning formulas, G. Harry McLaughlin's SMOG Grading does not directly measure the sentence length. Instead, it zeroes in on the word length in a selected passage. McLaughlin acknowledges that word and sentence length are the two linguistic measures which have the best predictive power for determining readability. However, McLaughlin argues that previous readability specialists have gen-

---

*Adapted from *The Technique of Clear Writing.* Copyright © 1972 by Robert Gunning. Used with permission.

erally overlooked or ignored the fact that semantic difficulty (word length) and syntactic difficulty (sentence length) interact. In effect, the sentence length of a passage correlates highly with the number of "hard" words (or what other specialists would call *unknown* or *polysyllabic* words).[22] Because of this correlation and because the number of sentences to be analyzed is fixed at 30, the SMOG Grade can be determined by counting only the number of words of three or more syllables, estimating that number's square root, and then adding 3 to the square root to obtain the approximate reading grade.

McLaughlin believes that 100 words is too small a sample. And so even though the SMOG formula eliminates the multiplication chore, it does require a 30-sentence sample, which is roughly 600 words. Thus, using this formula could pose a problem if the nurse is writing a brief fact sheet. But for many longer leaflets or pamphlets, the SMOG formula can be quite valuable.

McLaughlin's directions for SMOG Grading are as follows:

1. *Count 10 consecutive sentences near the beginning of the text to be assessed, 10 in the middle, and 10 near the end.* Count as a sentence any string of words ending with a period, question mark, or exclamation point.

2. *In the 30 selected sentences count every word of three or more syllables.* Any string of letters or numerals beginning and ending with a space or punctuation mark should be counted if you can distinguish at least three syllables when you read it aloud in context. If a polysyllabic word is repeated, count each repetition.

3. *Estimate the square root of the number of polysyllabic words counted.* This is done by taking the square root of the nearest perfect square. For example, if the count is 95, the nearest perfect square is 100, which yields a square root of 10. If the count lies roughly between two perfect squares, choose the lower number. For instance, if the count is 110, take the square root of 100 rather than that of 121.

4. *Add 3 to the approximate square root. This gives the SMOG Grade, which is the reading grade that a person must have reached if he is to understand fully the text assessed.*[23]*

As you can see in Exhibit 3.1, the results of SMOG Grading are similar to those obtained previously from the Fog Index. Academic, scientific, and professional journals are usually written at the "difficult" to "very

---

*Reprinted with permission of G. Harry McLaughlin and the International Reading Association.

Exhibit 3.1. SMOG grade and interpretation.

SMOG Grade	Level of Style	Typical Magazine Example
6 – 7	Very easy	Comics
8	Easy	Pulp fiction
9 – 10	Average	*Reader's Digest*
11 – 13	Fairly difficult	*Atlantic Monthly*
14 – 16	Difficult	Academic journals
17 – up	Very difficult	Scientific journals

difficult" level, whereas magazines of "average" readability are represented by the SMOG Grade (or grade level) of 9–10.

One other readability yardstick worth reviewing is called the *cloze* procedure.[24] It is another quick way to assess how appropriate your writing is for a selected population. Although a cloze score does not represent a grade or reading level, it can be especially valuable when you are uncertain about which of two (or more) pieces you have written is more readable for the target audience.

To prepare the pieces for testing, you systematically delete words from various passages. Then, each word omitted is replaced with the same 10-letter blank, no matter how long the deleted word may have been. Readers from the target audience are asked to supply the missing words. The writing sample that receives or "scores" the largest total of correctly filled-in words is judged more readable for the selected population.

FORMAT SELECTION

Although the point may be fairly obvious from the discussion so far, it is worth stressing here that the overall format that the nurse educator chooses for conveying client information is often crucial to the successful use of the material. To cite just one illustration, researchers Florence S. Downs and Virginia Fernbach found that the prenatal leaflet series entitled *You're Having a Baby* (sponsored by the Metropolitan Life Insurance Company in 1970) was not entirely successful with the audience for which it was intended. Since many of the clients did not register for prenatal care until their pregnancies were advanced, they were given several leaflets at once. But this practice defeated the purpose of the series, namely, to provide clients with small bits of information systematically. Downs and Fernbach argue that the progressive leaflet series format "may be more appropriate for middle-class women who tend to begin prenatal care earlier in their pregnancy."[25]

The interplay, therefore, between format, audience, purpose, and type of information that the nurse writer wants to convey is extremely important. A six-page pamphlet on routine wound care seems excessive in light of the amount of information normally given to the client. But the same size pamphlet may be quite an appropriate format to reinforce the enterostomal nurse therapist's discharge instructions to colostomy clients.

Here are some different formats that you can use effectively to communicate information to clients:

- *Instructional or Informational Sheets*. These are one-page (8½″ × 11″) or half-page sheets that give clients brief instructions on how to assume self-care responsibilities at home. Or they may inform clients about the nature of a diagnostic test that has been scheduled.
- *Leaflets*. These consist of one piece of paper, usually 8½″ × 11″, folded one or more times. Usually information is conveyed on all sides of the leaflet.
- *Pamphlets*. These are small, unbound publications, often up to 15 pages long.
- *Booklets*. These may be unbound or softbound publications over 15 pages.
- *Posters*. These are large written or printed charts that can be displayed publicly or used in client teaching situations.
- *Instructional or Informational Cards*. These are popular and useful for teaching clients about medication regimens or drug information. They may be as large as 4″ × 6″, but often they are small enough to fit in clients' wallets. National organizations also find wallet cards helpful in informing others about clients' health problems in an emergency situation.

GENERAL GUIDELINES FOR WRITING HEALTH EDUCATION MATERIALS

In light of our preliminary discussion of audience analysis, readability formulas, and format selection just completed, you should now be prepared to consider—and to apply to your own writing—the following general guidelines for writing health education materials.

Guideline 1
Survey a representative sample of clients to find out what baseline knowledge they have acquired about a selected health problem or

disease, what misconceptions they currently hold, and what they would like to learn about the problem. Downs and Fernbach recommend that "surveys of the actual population to which an information piece is to be directed be carried out before materials are developed."[26] In this way, it is possible to avoid unfounded biases on the part of those who prepare the health care materials concerning what the population does or does not know and what learning styles are best for a particular socioeconomic group.

Guideline 2

Define the audience or client population according to the factors already discussed under audience analysis: age, ethnicity, socioeconomic status, educational background, and physiological status. In general, the more heterogeneous the audience, the more difficult it will be to design and write health education materials especially for that population.

Guideline 3

Determine the focus or purpose of your educational material and which format best suits the audience's needs. Discharge instructions for parents whose child has had an appendectomy will focus on specific procedures or precautions that parents or family members should continue at home. The focus, then, is on informing parents how to continue the child's convalescent care. Since the information will not be complex, a one-page instruction sheet would probably be the best format to use (Exhibit 3.2).

On the other hand, if the purpose of the written information is to give parents a background review of the rooms, mealtimes, lounge facilities, and routines of the pediatric unit, a more extensive pamphlet of perhaps six pages or so would be a more appropriate format. Of course, the complexity and amount of information have to be considered here.

Guideline 4

Assess your clients' reading level. You can do this informally when they complete other patient-related information when they are admitted to an acute care institution or when they make the initial contact with an ambulatory care facility. If the audience has difficulty with admission materials written at the tenth grade level, you can be fairly sure that health care materials you write will need to be written at a somewhat lower level.

You can also assess the audience's reading level by asking people to rate two previously prepared and graded passages, either by the cloze procedure described earlier in this chapter or by subjective analysis (Which did you like better? Why? Was one easier to understand?). Both these techniques are helpful in assessing the general reading level of an

Exhibit 3.2. One-page instruction sheet.

AFTER AN APPENDECTOMY . . .
HOME CARE INSTRUCTIONS FOR YOUR CHILD

1. Keep your child quiet at home until the doctor checks him or her. Reading, watching TV, drawing or coloring, and playing card games are some quiet things your child might like to do.
2. Your child will probably be able to go back to school after the checkup. He or she should stay out of gym class for at least 4 weeks — or until your doctor says it's OK.
3. Check your child's incision daily for
   - Redness or swelling
   - Drainage or bleeding
   - Separation or opening
   - More pain around the incision
   - Any other stomach pain
4. If your child has a dressing, change it every day or as often as your doctor tells you. Call him or her right away if you notice any increased drainage or bad smell from the incision.
   - IMPORTANT: Wash your hands well *before* and *after* you change your child's dressing.
5. Let your child eat the foods he or she feels like eating. It is normal for your child not to eat as much as usual when first coming home.
   - IMPORTANT: Have your child drink *at least* 6 4-oz glasses of liquid every day. Don't let your child get constipated so that he or she can't have a bowel movement.
6. Your child may take a sponge bath or shower. Your doctor will tell you when it's OK for a tub bath.
7. Call your doctor's office when you get home today to make an appointment for your child's checkup on _____ .
8. Additional instructions: _____
   _____
   _____
   _____

---

audience with specific learning needs you are trying to address—for example, adult insulin-dependent diabetics or young adults who have multiple sclerosis.

Guideline 5

Research the literature to discover the most current, accurate information available on your topic. The importance of using accurate, up-to-date information should be self-evident. Today's clients entering the health care system have become quite "consumer oriented" and feel they have the right to the best health information possible. If the educational materials you write reflect this philosophy, readers will be more likely to respect them as reliable information sources.

Guideline 6
Consult with local authorities, such as nurse specialists and physicians, to gather their input as well as to have them critique what you have written. In their article "Health Education Literature for Parents of Handicapped Children," researchers Ivan Barry Pless and Betty Satterwhite reaffirm previous studies showing that parent information booklets are more likely to be read and respected if they are prepared by "prestigeful authorities."[27] And so nurses who prepare and write health education materials should give credit to those experts who review, critique, or contribute to the preparation of the information. Appropriate credit for a pamphlet on cast care for home-going orthopedic clients might appear as "Prepared by L. Jones, R.N., M.S.N., Orthopedic Clinical Nurse Specialist, in collaboration with F. Roberts, M.D., Chief of Orthopedic Surgery at Memorial Hospital" or as "Written by R. White, R.N., with the assistance of the Staff Nurses of 5-East." Giving credit to the experts and authorities who prepare the educational materials not only makes the health care consumer more respectful of the information but also acknowledges the authorities' help and preparation time. Furthermore, any other health care providers who use the information in client teaching know whom to contact if there are questions they cannot answer.

Guideline 7
Write directly to the client or to his or her family (or significant other). In general, parents will not respond favorably to information that refers to their child as "the patient." Clients read health information for practical, personal reasons; they are concerned about *their* body, *their* lifestyle, and being able to manage *their* problems. So, in writing directly to them, use *you* and *your*. The tone you convey with the second person will be less formal, more conversational, and more meaningful to the audience.

Guideline 8
Based on data gathered from your surveys, write about what clients and their families *need* to know to take care of themselves or understand their health problem as well as what they would *like* to know. In his previously cited article for *Clinical Pediatrics,* Scanlon explains that he addressed the issue of what parents would *like* to know about innocent murmurs by asking them: "What kind of questions would you ask a physician if he told you that your child had an 'innocent' or 'functional' murmur?"[28] Although it might not be possible to cover all the points clients would like us to, certainly those mentioned most frequently could be included.

Guideline 9

Organize the information content in a logical sequence to avoid confusion. Delete whatever detracts from the focus or purpose of your message. Often, a brief topical outline helps you arrange the progression of information into a logical order so that neither you nor your prospective audience will become confused. Reading aloud what you have written may help you spot errors in logic as well as clarify the message you want to convey.

Guideline 10

Choose appropriate language. Specifically, avoid using medical or nursing terms unless such technical terms are absolutely necessary to the successful meaning or understanding of the material. When you believe it is essential to employ a word a client may not know, be sure to define it within the context of the writing, taking care "not to distort the true meaning of terms when simplifying for a lay audience."[29]

Guideline 11

Prepare your materials to meet your audience's previously assessed reading level. Consider that writing geared to levels above the tenth grade may not always be effectively understood, even if many in your target audience can read at the twelfth grade level. The stress of illness may hamper some clients' ability to comprehend written directions and instructions.

Consider, too, other factors that can greatly influence the readability of a pamphlet. Besides using short, familiar words and writing short sentences and paragraphs, you may be most effective if you vary your sentences so that occasionally a compact and incisive sentence appears in the midst of somewhat longer sentences. Using large or varied print size, boldface type, illustrations, headings and subheadings, and itemizations or lists will also vary the page format and give your writing more appeal.

Incorporating well-designed illustrations into your writing deserves special mention. Realistic yet tasteful illustrations can gain your clients' attention and may encourage them to read your instruction sheet or pamphlet. Purdue University's Steven E. Pauley recommends that writers choose illustrations as carefully as the words they employ, since the purpose of illustrations is to capture visually—and thus enhance—key points within a written message.[30] Illustrations or figures should be integrated within the writing at logical, convenient places. They should not precede the relevant written information but instead follow the discussion of an important point in the text. If you place an illustration in your writing *before* you explain or discuss it, your readers may wonder why it is there.

Guideline 12
Obtain a final critique of content by submitting a clean copy of your rough draft to clinical experts currently practicing in the field. Such experts could include nurse educators, clinical nurse specialists, physicians, or staff nurses with advanced expertise in the area about which you are writing. Review their comments and suggestions, and incorporate them as needed to produce the most authoritative educational reference material possible.

Guideline 13
Evaluate the preliminary draft by having a sample audience population read the information and complete a questionnaire based on the content, readability, and ease with which it was understood. This pilot testing will enable you to spot difficult areas and can give you ideas on how to revise the writing.

Guideline 14
After you prepare your final draft, find at least one person with good editorial skills to help you proofread for punctuation, spelling, or mechanical errors. Glaring errors detract from the overall credibility of the material; they may cause miscommunication on the part of the professional educator or the client. Careful proofreading is a painstaking process, but the error-free product indicates careful and professional work.

Guideline 15
As a final check before the information is printed, answer these questions:

- Is the purpose of the material clear?
- Is the language appropriate for the audience level?
- Are the sentences clear?
- Is the content correct?
- Is the format appealing?
- Has anything been omitted?

WRITING CLEAR INSTRUCTIONS AND READABLE INFORMATION

Nurses in most clinical areas are often involved in writing succinct, easy-to-understand instructional fact sheets to use in teaching or reinforcing self-care activities. These printed instructions enable clients to have a ready reference source so that they can actively participate in their own rehabilitation, either inside or outside of the health care facility. Types of instructional or informational sheets the nurse prepares include discharge instructions, medication instructions and precautions, and specific information on how to carry out therapeutic procedures such as colostomy irrigations, tracheotomy care, and the like.

Because there is an abundance of health information available to instruct clients on such topics as hypertension, chronic obstructive pulmonary disease, and diabetes, the nurse may not need to write instructions related to these topics. But the nurse must know how to choose the materials wisely, according to the principles of effective writing, and how to evaluate the success of the materials, based on the audience's comprehension.

On the other hand, the nurse may find that no commercially printed health information adequately meets the needs of the agency's client population. This situation may be due to the unique composition of the audience, to agency protocols, to nursing preferences, or to the medical regimen. In this instance, the nurse will find that specially prepared instructions geared specifically for the audience, taking into account nursing, agency, and medical preferences, will be more suitable than commercially prepared information. In addition, such tailor-made instructions should be less confusing to clients.

For written instructions to be effective, they must be read, understood, and remembered by clients. Thus, the nurse writer must consciously apply the principles of audience analysis and judiciously use readability formulas to assess the appropriateness of the instruction sheet. Furthermore, clients will be more likely to remember the instructions if the written information reinforces prior oral messages. And so nurses who use in their *oral* explanations both an organizational plan and terminology similar to those that occur in the *written* information avoid the potential problem of confusing clients who look at the instruction sheet once they are home. Clients should not experience discrepancies between oral and written instructions.

One of the most important points to consider when writing client instruction sheets is how much detail to include. The most reliable method of determining this is to do a needs assessment of what the audience would like to know before going home or before feeling ready to assume self-care responsibilities. Because instruction sheets are often a combination of information and instructions, providing just the right degree of detail can be crucial to successful communication of the material. The clients' comprehension of the material can be tested by asking them to verbalize the instructions or return the demonstration. Such informal factors, as well as surveying the sample client population after it has used and assessed the instruction sheet, should give you data about the correct proportion of detail to incorporate in the future.

Guidelines for Writing Instructions

Here are some useful guidelines for writing effective instructions for clients. You will notice that they follow naturally from the 15 general guidelines we previously discussed.

Guideline 1
Determine the audience's level and the basic information clients need to know to carry out the instructions properly. If there is a great deal of basic information to convey before clients can carry out the process or procedure, you may want to write two different client-teaching aids. For example, one might be an informational fact sheet on sigmoid colostomies; the other could focus exclusively on the steps clients take in irrigating the colostomy.

Guideline 2
Determine just how complex the instructions are. In general, the more complicated the instructions, the greater the necessity of breaking them down into discrete steps. If you actually perform the procedure yourself, you can determine exactly how many separate steps the process has. There is a considerable difference between (1) preparing written reinforcement instructions for the parent who will be performing tracheotomy care and (2) writing follow-up instructions for middle class adults for routine incision care. Because the instructions for the first procedure are going to be more involved, they will have to be broken down into numerous distinct steps to be better understood by the audience.

Guideline 3
Keep your style clear and concise by using relatively short sentences (10–15 words), the active voice, and action verbs. Avoid passive constructions such as "The insulin is to be given. . . ." or "The wound must be irrigated every day." Instead, choose the more dynamic imperative form: "Irrigate the wound every day with a solution of . . . ." or "Give your insulin in the morning about 30 minutes before you eat your breakfast."

Guideline 4
Consider whether there is a fixed, sequential order or a flexible order of choice for the process, procedure, or set of instructions you are writing.

Decide exactly what is to be done, as well as where, when, how, and by whom. A fixed order means that there is essentially only one way of arranging the steps in the sequence: step 1 must be completed before step 2, step 2 before step 3, and so on. Order of choice means that there is no fixed sequence; the writer tries to organize the instructions according to some reasonable principle (chronological and topical are two possibilities).

Guideline 5
Use illustrations wisely. Since poor drawings or pictures may confuse the reader, do not use them if they do not complement or clarify your written instructions.

Discharge Instructions

Written discharge instructions are frequently used in acute care settings to document patient education and discharge teaching. As Sylvia L. Burkey points out in her recent *Supervisor Nurse* article entitled "An Audit Outcome: Home Going Instructions," written discharge instructions are especially valuable for coordinating nurses' teaching activities with physicians' health care prescriptions.[31]

The two types of discharge instructions most commonly used in hospitals are (1) general instruction sheets, often set up in a semistructured format, that can be adapted for a variety of health education needs and (2) instructions related to specific health problems, illnesses, or surgeries.

Burkey describes a semistructured discharge instruction sheet containing information on diet, activity, wound care, medications, and follow-up care. Although the physician is responsible for the home-going health education content of the instructions, the nurse translates the instructions, teaching according to the patient's needs, and often writing the physician's instructions according to the patient's comprehension. "The nurse may re-state the instructions in lay terms (as if writing a letter to the patient),"[32] states Burkey. The comparison between writing instructions and writing a letter really is appropriate, for informal letters are usually easy to understand, friendly, and nonthreatening.

Exhibit 3.3 shows a semistructured discharge instruction sheet that physicians at one institution use to document their discharge health prescriptions. The nurse follows up by reinforcing the prescriptions, clarifying instructions, teaching special procedures (wound care, for instance), and teaching and reinforcing printed home care instructions. And finally, Exhibit 3.4 shows home care or discharge instructions written especially for the posthysterectomy patient.

PEDIATRIC DISCHARGE INSTRUCTIONS
The Barberton Citizens Hospital

Discharge instructions for: _____

Diagnosis: _____

☐ Diet
_____ As tolerated
_____ Encourage fluids first 2-3 days to 4-5 8 oz.
glasses per day. Do not allow child to become
constipated.
_____ Special _____
_____

☐ Bathing
_____ Shower _____ Tub _____ Sponge

Incision Care
Always wash hands before and after checking
dressing
1. Check dressing daily for increased drainage.
2. Change dressing _____
3. Clean incision at dressing change with
_____

4. Notify Physician immediately if any of the
following are apparent:
a. redness
b. increased swelling
c. drainage or bleeding
d. opening of incision
e. increased pain around incision

☐ Medicines
If any increase in pain or fever occurs, call the
doctor.
_____ Tylenol or aspirin may be used for pain or
fever as directed.
_____ Prescriptions: _____
_____
_____
_____

☐ Printed home care instructions given and
explained.

☐ Activity
_____ Keep child in house until seen by doctor
_____ No school until _____
_____ Gradual return to normal activity
_____ No strenuous activity until checked by
physician
_____ No Gym until _____
_____ Other _____
_____
_____

☐ Extremity Care
1. Check your child's fingers/toes several times a
day. They should be warm and pink. Your child
should be able to move his/her fingers/toes
without too much discomfort. Press fingers/toes
gently. The nail beds should appear white and
return to normal pink color when pressure is
released. Note whether or not the fingers/toes
are swollen. If you have problems with any of
these, call your doctor.
2. If any numbness, tingling, or burning occurs, call
your doctor.
3. Elevate the extremity on a pillow when sitting or
in bed. This will prevent swelling.
4. Check dressing daily for increased drainage.

☐ Additional instructions: _____
_____
_____
_____
_____
_____

Please call my office _____ and make an appointment to see me in _____ days/weeks.

_____ M.D./D.O.

I have received and understand the above instructions

_____
Parent or Responsible Person & Relationship

#3256 (10 79)
Patient copy (white) Med Record (canary)

PATIENT COPY

Exhibit 3.3. Semistructured discharge instruction sheet.

Exhibit 3.4. Home care instructions.

HOW TO TAKE CARE OF YOURSELF
AFTER YOUR HYSTERECTOMY

YOUR SLEEP/REST
NEEDS

1. Get plenty of sleep and rest. It is normal for you to get tired easily when you get home. You will probably feel like lying down or taking an afternoon nap, especially during your first week out of the hospital.

YOUR ACTIVITIES

2. *Gradually* return to your normal routine that you followed before your surgery. Don't lift anything heavy for 4 to 6 weeks.
This means . . .
•No laundry baskets of wet clothes
•No infants over 15 lb
•No bags of groceries
•No heavy packages or household tools

Avoid heavy cleaning chores for 4 weeks.
This means . . .
•No vacuuming
•No floor scrubbing
•No window washing
Light dusting and "straightening up" are OK. Do not go on long shopping trips or drive for 4 weeks.

Do not have intercourse (sex) for 4 weeks or until your doctor says it's OK.

YOUR INCISION

Tell your doctor about any change in your incision—swelling, pain, or bad-smelling drainage. Keep the incision clean.
SPECIAL INSTRUCTIONS: _____

YOUR BATH

You may shower when you feel up to it. But ask your doctor when it's all right to take a tub bath.

YOUR MEDICINE

If your doctor has prescribed any medicine for you, take it as he ordered. If the medicine bothers you, call him. *Don't stop taking it without telling him!* He may change the medicine, or he may tell you that it's OK to stop taking it.

YOUR DIET

Drink at least 6 to 8 glasses of water or juice every day. Try to include two servings of fruit and two servings of vegetables in your diet every day. Plenty of liquids, fruits, and vegetables will help you from getting constipated or straining to have a bowel movement. Otherwise, eat the foods you like, unless you're on a special diet.

WHEN TO CALL
YOUR DOCTOR

Call your doctor . . .
•If you run a fever (over 101°) for more than 24 hours
•If you notice any change in passing your urine—such as having to go frequently, blood in your urine, or a burning feeling
•If you should have over three saturated pads a day of *bright red bleeding*
It is normal to have slight to moderate amounts of dark red or brown drainage for several weeks.

140

WRITING ABOUT MEDICATIONS

Preparing or selecting appropriately written drug information and instructions has become an important part of the nurse's teaching activities. Probably the appearance of patient package inserts, required for all oral contraceptives since 1970, has provided the greatest impetus to the use of written drug information as an adjunct to teaching activities. Louis A. Morris and Jerome A. Halperin's review of the literature on the effectiveness of written drug information indicates that some aspects of client failure to take prescribed medications (noncompliance) are "certainly due to the failure of traditional modes of communication." They further comment that "written instructions can serve to enhance the probability that important information can be presented, and will be attended to, understood, accepted, and recalled."[33] Of course, clear instructions and open communication between the health care provider and the client do not guarantee that compliance will occur. Dorothy L. Smith, author of *Medication Guide for Patient Counseling,* agrees that written instructions may foster compliance by providing clients with the basic information they need to manage effectively their drug regimens. She cautions, however, that written instructions should not replace oral communication with the client.[34] Indeed, the value of written drug information is similar to that of most other health education materials prepared for a selected client population—to reinforce, to supplement, to serve as a permanent resource to the nurse educator's teaching session with the client.

Several formats are available for written drug information. Some useful styles include instructional stickers pasted on the bottle or package, checklists of precautions and side effects, folded or unfolded wallet-size cards, handouts the size of index cards, patient package inserts, one- or two-page instruction sheets or leaflets, and pamphlets and booklets.[35] Programmed instruction has even been adapted successfully to teach clients about the drug Warfarin, an oral anticoagulant.[36]

In some instances, the type of format has been closely associated with different groups of health professionals. For example, pharmacists have been the primary group of health care providers to employ checklists fairly successfully. Although stickers may be the easiest way for pharmacists to inform clients of necessary instructions and the like, checklists give them more flexibility because special instructions can be written directly on the sheet. Nurses might also find a checklist format valuable in selected situations. But nurses traditionally have used the drug card or one-page instruction sheet or leaflet, perhaps because the amount of information that can be included on the card or handout seems to suit most clients' learning needs.

Basically, the 15 general guidelines for writing health education materials that were presented earlier in this chapter apply to the writing of drug-related information and instructions. We need, however, to single out and review *four points* here that are essential to the successful writing and comprehension of drug information.

First, as with every other kind of written health information, you should analyze the client population to determine its informational needs. Ask yourself exactly what information clients need in order to take their medicines safely and effectively.

Second, you should include clear, meaningful illustrations when they will add to the comprehensibility of the written instructions. Illustrations also contribute significantly to the appeal and popularity of the material. For instance, one recent study comparing two different inserts for oral contraceptives reveals that clients preferred the booklet with pictures to the nonillustrated booklet.[37] And Smith's 1977 *Medication Guide* is worth looking at, for it incorporates several clear drawings to illustrate the instillation of eye drops, ear drops, nose drops, and vaginal creams. The calendars and diagrams that she uses to clarify oral contraceptive dosage schedules are also well done because they enhance the written instructions.

Exhibit 3.5. Drug information handout.

WHAT YOU SHOULD KNOW ABOUT . . .
YOUR HIGH BLOOD PRESSURE MEDICINE!

You are taking a high blood pressure medicine called ＿＿＿＿＿＿. It will lower your blood pressure by increasing the size of your body's blood vessels. And when the blood vessels get bigger, the pressure inside of them is *less*. And that's definitely good for *you!* *Less* pressure inside the blood vessels means that *your* blood pressure will be lower. One thing you must remember—*no matter how good you feel,* you must take your medicine *every day* to keep your pressure down!

One of the side effects of your medicine is called *postural hypotension*. This means that when you change position quickly, you may feel lightheaded or dizzy. This might occur when you . . .

- Stand up suddenly
- Get out of bed too fast
- Bend over quickly

You should move *slowly* to help relieve the dizziness or lightheaded feeling. If this feeling occurs frequently (say, more than twice a day), call the nurses at the clinic.

Your medicine may also cause your heart to beat faster. Sometimes it may make you feel hot or warm or flushed. If these things cause you problems, tell your nurse.

IMPORTANT: *Do not stop taking your medicine without calling the nurses at the clinic! Remember—we want to help you keep your pressure down!*

CLINIC PHONE NUMBER ＿＿＿＿＿＿   YOUR BLOOD PRESSURE MEDICINE

YOUR NURSE ＿＿＿＿＿＿＿＿   DOSAGE ＿＿＿＿＿＿＿＿

SPECIAL INSTRUCTIONS

Third, by writing concise, simple instructions, you can help all clients—but especially the elderly—comply with their drug regimens. Morris and Halperin cite a British study which showed that elderly clients receiving short, simple instructions on drug cards complied far better than those in the control group.[38] Exhibit 3.5 is a drug information handout prepared especially for elderly hypertension clients at an outpatient clinic.

Fourth, you should be specific and highlight important instructions that are essential to the client's drug regimen. You may want to use large type, underline the information, indent and list it, or repeat it at certain times on the instructional sheet. Any method that sets it off or calls attention to it can be used. Examples of information to emphasize include not discontinuing the drug without calling the health agency, taking all the prescribed drug, taking the drug with or without food, and taking the drug even though the client feels well. Headings such as "Important" and "Precautions" also signal significant points. To be sure, you want to achieve a balance between alerting the client and unduly frightening the client. But as Evalee Keck Leeper so aptly states, "In writing about medication, we must overcome the prevailing casual attitude toward the giving or taking of drugs."[39]

WRITING NURSE-CLIENT CONTRACTS

The use of written nurse-client contracts has been firmly established in the nursing literature for the past decade. Essentially, a nurse-client contract is a nonlegal, goal-setting agreement between the client and the health care provider. It is based on the assumption that the nurse and the client are partners—with different but equal responsibilities—in the management of the client's health status. A contract, then, is a viable tool that the professional nurse can use to help the client reach mutually agreeable goals or target behaviors to stabilize or improve his or her health status.

But a contract is more than a tool. It is also a methodological process based on these seven steps:

1. Collecting baseline data
2. Discussing nurse-client expectations of each other
3. Formulating mutually agreeable goals
4. Establishing the contract that delineates client and nurse responsibilities
5. Coordinating the contract with staff and significant others

6. Evaluating the contract in light of the client's progress toward the goals
7. Terminating the contract if the goals are met, or recontracting if they need modification[40]

Using nurse-client contracts offers several advantages. First, contracting requires that clients take a more active role in their care, becoming "activists who choose the options they can realistically follow, rather than passive victims of the health care system."[41] Because contracting emphasizes the clients' participation in their care, Professors Steckel and Swain found that compliance was enhanced in those hypertensive outpatients for whom the contracting process was an integral part of the therapeutic regimen. No clients dropped out of the contract group; but about 8% dropped out of the routine clinic care group, and about 36% dropped out of the group that received education and counseling without the contracting component. Steckel and Swain conclude, therefore, that "treatment intervention and contracting for a return visit can influence continued participation in clinic care; however, education and routine care, without contracting, is not an effective means of getting patients to continue treatment."[42]

Furthermore, in her *Nursing Outlook* article entitled "It's the Patient's Problem—and Decision," Karyl K. Blair points out that one of the most important advantages in using nurse-client contracts is *not* giving clients services they don't want or are not yet ready for. The contracting process can help staff members manage their time more productively: "We no longer use hundreds of nurse-hours trying to guess what the patient wants or . . . will accept as a possible solution. . . . We also recognize the fruitlessness of using several hours of nursing time trying to convince a family to work on a health problem that the family does not see as a problem."[43]

Finally, the contracting process not only specifies the client's participant role in self-care activities but also clarifies the nurse's role (such as providing coordinating functions, counseling, teaching, or therapeutic services). And defining who is responsible for what activities is especially important as more members of the health care team become involved in the client's care. Knowing where the responsibility lies for the coordinated activities also makes it much easier to write the care plan.

Now, even though current nursing literature shows how successful contracting can be in a variety of situations and settings as well as for clients of various ages, there are some clients who probably will not benefit from contracting. Some clients might not want to be more active in their own health care. Others might possess only "minimal cognitive skills."[44] Still others might not be capable of making decisions about their treatment because of a current health crisis.

Components of Nurse-Client Contracts

Essentially, three components make up a good nurse-client contract: (1) short-term goals, (2) long-term goals, and (3) a reinforcement or reward system. Goals are often referred to as *target behaviors* because this term more aptly expresses the fact that a goal is an observable activity toward which the client and nurse are striving. Goals should be stated in behavioral terms to allow all parties involved to understand clearly what is being sought.

Since contracting is based on the principles of behavior modification, the reinforcement or reward system becomes an integral part of nurse-client contracting. Reinforcement, according to William J. DeRisi and George Butz, provides "consequences for behavior in order to increase the likelihood that it will occur again or more frequently than in the past. This usually involves giving something, including attention, objects of special value, or privileges." The reinforcing event, then, is the "opportunity to engage in some activity that is highly valued."[45]

Reinforcers are generally of two types—social (often expressions of approval) or tangible (often concrete items, such as money, food, or new clothes, whose reception depends on achieving the goal). While nurses do not usually dispense tangible reinforcers to clients, they do have many opportunities to give valuable social reinforcers. Or they may help negotiate tangible reinforcers between clients and other family members, as Professors Wang and Watson describe in a recent article about the contracting process between a 12-year-old girl and her father to lose weight.[46] Interestingly, when nurses gave clients in one setting the opportunity to choose tangible reinforcers, the most frequently chosen rewards were "lottery tickets, money, books, magazines, and time with the health care provider. Some of the rewards did not cost anything, and those that did averaged $1."[47]

Reinforcers should be chosen with care, whether they consist of praise or attention, valuable objects, or privileges. They should be meaningful to the client—you will need to seek reliable feedback here—and readily deliverable.

Guidelines for Writing Nurse-Client Contracts

Written nurse-client contracts are generally not long, nor are they difficult to write. The value of a written contract (as opposed to an oral one) is that it gives clients something tangible to refer to in an acute care setting or to take home with them from an outpatient facility. Written contracts also help improve compliance. One research study recently demonstrated that written contracts markedly increased juvenile diabetics' compliance with urine testing as compared to compliance when the same goals were set orally.[48] The following eight guidelines will help you to write effective nurse-client contracts.

Guideline 1

With the client, determine the short-term and long-term goals or target behaviors that you want to achieve. Focus on behavior—measurable, observable activity—not on those elements, such as attitudes, values, or feelings, that cannot be measured directly. Use specific, concrete action verbs that clearly state what you and the client want him or her to do, perform, or achieve:

- To lose 5 lb
- To walk the length of the hall twice a day
- To jog 1 mile every morning
- To eat fresh fruits and vegetables between meals

Guideline 2

When the long-term goal (often referred to as the final outcome or terminal behavior) is complex and consists of several more easily achieved goals, organize them in order of increasing difficulty. For instance, weekly goals for an adolescent girl contracting to lose weight were to

1. Eat sitting down in the dining room only
2. Return her utensils to the table and put her hands on her lap after taking a mouthful until the mouthful is swallowed
3. Eat only fresh fruits, celery, and carrots between meals
4. Eat only in the presence of others
5. Eat one normal serving from each food item on the table
6. Eat no food between meals[49]

Guideline 3

Since positively stated goals have a better chance of motivating people to help themselves than do negatively stated goals, write them in positive terms from the client's viewpoint. Usually, the words "I will" followed by the specific action verb convey the positive framework to prompt the appropriate target behavior.

Guideline 4

Decide how the client can reward himself or herself or be rewarded by others for achieving his or her goal. Because rewards or reinforcers must be meaningful to the client, ask him or her to identify those things that serve as strong motivators for achieving the target behavior. DeRisi and Butz believe that the contract should also state exactly how and when the reinforcer will be delivered.[50] Just as it may be helpful to rank goals in order of increasing difficulty, so also can reinforcers be ranked in order of increasing worth—from having some free time during the day to read a novel (as a way of reinforcing the decision not to eat between meals) to taking a vacation (as a reward for losing 50 lb).

Guideline 5

Determine client responsibilities and nurse responsibilities, and express them clearly in the contract. An "If . . . then" conditional statement may be used to spell out both parties' responsibilities, or it may be implied. The client situation that follows illustrates how the "If . . . then" statement expresses the client's and the nurse's responsibilities.

> Mr. Glenn Howard is a 45-year-old diabetic with moderate learning disabilities. Because of his basic personality and his difficulty in comprehending health concepts related to his newly diagnosed condition, he has been refusing to eat supper. As a result, he has had significant hypoglycemic reactions around 10 PM for the past five evenings. The diabetic nurse educator's attempts to teach him about his problem have not succeeded. The nurse notes, however, that Mr. Howard is devoted to checkers and is always asking nursing personnel to play a game with him. The nurse decides that contracting might be a viable way of getting Mr. Howard to comply with his diet, with a game of checkers serving as a powerful reinforcer. When the contract idea is brought up, he is very enthusiastic. Not only can he understand the simplified contract but also he can articulate a simple goal with the nurse—"to feel good again at night before I go to bed." The reinforcer gives Mr. Howard the motivation to comply with the dietary regimen.

The nurse educator in the preceding situation wrote the contract with Mr. Howard using the conditional statement: "If Mr. Howard eats all his supper within 45 minutes of getting his tray, then the nurse will spend 15 uninterrupted minutes at bedtime playing a game of checkers with him." Notice that the first segment gives the client's behavior or responsibilities, whereas the second segment gives the nurse's responsibilities. In this case, too, the nurse is part of the reward system.

Guideline 6

Should you prefer not to write contracts with conditional statements, use instead a two-column format (see Exhibit 3.6) that lists the specific activities or duties of, first, the client and, second, the nurse. Although an "If . . . then" conditional statement *may* be implied in *some* circumstances

Exhibit 3.6. Contract in two-column format.

NURSE-CLIENT CONTRACT

LONG-TERM GOAL:

SHORT-TERM GOAL:

REWARD/REINFORCER:

NURSE RESPONSIBILITIES   *CLIENT RESPONSIBILITIES*

Nurse Signature/Date	Client Signature/Date

Family Member/Date

TO BE EVALUATED:

---

between the responsibilities listed under *client* and those listed under *nurse,* the overall intent here is to differentiate what the parties will do to help the client achieve long- and short-term health goals. Thus, the nurse's responsibilities for providing coordinating functions or therapeutic services are not dependent on the client's behavioral activities.

In this case, too, specific reinforcers may lie more within the client's domain. For example, the client may have the option of modifying his or her activity or of receiving extra pain medication after uncomfortable therapeutic regimens such as dressing changes. When the contract is written so that both parties' responsibilities are *separately* defined, the reinforcing or rewarding agent may be the attainment of the long- or short-term goal itself. Many nurses feel more comfortable with this type of contractual agreement since they participate less directly in the reinforcer system.

Guideline 7
Date and sign the contract. If a family member or significant other is providing reinforcement or rewards for the client, then that person should also sign. While bonus clauses for "sustained or exceptional performance"[51] are often helpful, penalty statements that indicate the conse-

quences if the specific behavior is not performed should be avoided, for penalties or punishments are not nearly as successful (as are positive reinforcers) in motivating people.

Guideline 8
Indicate the evaluation or review date and, if necessary, the means by which the contract will be evaluated. Evaluation is an integral part of nurse-client contracts. Indeed, it is only by evaluating what has occurred that both parties know whether the contract was successful or needs to be revised. As one nurse educator explains, the means of evaluation for ambulatory clients may be "a phone call, a mailed note, a return visit, or a meeting with a person other than the nurse."[52]

SUMMARY

Today's professional nurses are becoming increasingly involved in selecting, using, evaluating, and even composing written health care information for their clients. Indeed, nurses at many agencies often cooperate in designing and writing client education materials to better meet the needs of their specific audience. In focusing on writing readable health information for the client, we can profitably consider seven important topic areas.

First, there is audience analysis. Successful writers in *all* fields never lose sight of the people for whom they are writing. Writers who have analyzed their audience and have taken into account its special problems, concerns, and needs do a more effective job of conveying their message.

Once we have analyzed the audience, the critical element to consider is readability. Just how easy is it for the audience to read and understand the written information? Several readability formulas have been developed to help writers estimate the reading difficulty of written materials.

Format selection, the third topic area, is based on the premise that the overall format that the nurse educator chooses for conveying client information is often crucial to the successful use of the material.

Next, it is useful to know and apply the 15 general guidelines for writing health education materials. These general guidelines can help writers through the planning, writing, and revising stages for a variety of materials.

Writing clear instructions and readable information, the fifth topic area, includes five specific guidelines for writing effective instructions for clients. Moreover, written discharge instructions are frequently used in acute care settings to document patient education and discharge teaching.

Writing about medications, the sixth topic area, includes four points that are essential to the successful writing and comprehension of drug information.

And writing nurse-client contracts, the last topic area, explains contracting as both a viable tool and a methodological process that the professional nurse can use to help the client reach mutually agreeable goals to stabilize or improve his or her health status.

EXERCISES

1. Rewrite the following sentences from client education materials to make them *more* readable. The first three sentences might appear in a booklet on cast care, the last two sentences in a leaflet on respiratory care.

   a. Maintain adequate elevation of the extremity above the level of the heart, to prevent edema.

   b. Certain symptoms may appear that may suggest that the cast is constricting the extremity, such as inability to move digits, excessive pain, discolored nail beds, or unusual numbness or tingling.

   c. Exercise the fingers continually to improve circulation, keep edema minimal, and maintain proper functioning.

   d. The emphasis on drinking sufficient water is to facilitate the loosening of secretions, thus making it easier to expectorate mucus and eliminating a breeding place for bacteria.

   e. Paced pursed-lip breathing exercises will be explained by the nurse, as this technique helps to rid the lungs of carbon dioxide and therefore diminishes the number of episodes of shortness of breath.

2. Read carefully the following informational fact sheet given to clients at a large urban outpatient clinic to prepare them for an upper gastrointestinal examination. Most of the clients are Spanish-speaking, have less than a tenth grade education, and are between the ages of 16 and 50.

   Dear Client:

   Your physician has ordered a series of examinations of your gastrointestinal system. They are to be started tomorrow morning. As a result, you are to have only a light evening meal tonight, and then only water until midnight. After midnight, you will not receive anything orally, nor will you receive anything for breakfast. You are to be NPO until the testing sessions are considered terminated by the radiologist. Chewing gum and smoking are also prohibited until the examination is completed.

In the Radiology Department you will receive a flavored barium beverage that is not too unpleasant to take. The radiologist will fluoroscope your gastrointestinal system, including an x-ray of your stomach and duodenum at this time. When the examination is completed, you will be returned to the unit and will be permitted to have nourishment according to the diet previously prescribed by the physician.

If you have any questions concerning this examination, please do not hesitate to ask the nurse.

First, using the Gunning Fog Index, compute the readability (grade level) of this informational fact sheet. Is it possible to use the SMOG formula to determine the passage's readability? Second, write a 200-word critique of the informational fact sheet, citing both strengths and weaknesses. Finally, rewrite the fact sheet to improve its readability and its appeal to the audience for which it was intended.

3. Use McLaughlin's SMOG formula to analyze the readability of three or four commercially prepared booklets or leaflets on a specific disease or health problem—for example, diabetes, hypertension, or chronic obstructive lung disease. Consider analyzing the booklets and pamphlets from the American Heart Association, for they range from "very easy" to "fairly difficult."

4. According to Judith Petrello ("Your Patients Hear You, But Do They Understand?" *RN,* 39 [February 1976], 37–39), nurses at a large medical center hospital found the following words to be confusing for their patients. For each word, provide an alternative term or phrase that could make the meaning more understandable.

- Abscess
- Acute
- Compress
- Culture
- Fasting
- Hematocrit
- Hematoma
- Impaction
- Secretions
- Suction
- Tendon
- Traction

5. Read Deborah Vandewater's article, "Laryngectomee Leaflet," in *The Canadian Nurse,* 73 (August 1977), 48–50. Then complete the following activities:

   a. Determine the readability of the leaflet by using the Fog Index and the SMOG formula. How closely do the two grade levels correlate?

   b. Select one or two passages and use the cloze procedure to assess the passages' readability for another professional nurse, an allied health professional (such as an occupational therapist), and an ancillary employee (such as a unit secretary). What conclusions do you draw from your preliminary study?

c. Evaluate the appropriateness and visual impact of the two illustrations in the leaflet. Seek input from those who participated in your preliminary study.

d. What specific suggestions and techniques would you discuss with another professional who wants to use this tool with a client who will be undergoing a laryngectomy? Write a summary of your recommendations and discuss them with your class.

6. Read Lois S. Dwyer and Florence G. Fralin's article, "Simplified Meal Planning for Hard-to-Teach Patients," in *American Journal of Nursing,* 74 (April 1974), 664–665. The authors describe the use of a colorful, easy-to-read chart to instruct clients with impaired vision or poor reading abilities about their special diets. Develop a similar chart for clients with poor reading skills to teach them about their long-term health problems, such as hypertension or arthritis.

7. You are a staff nurse on a 40-bed general surgery unit. Since up to 25% of the clients on the unit are admitted for elective cholecystectomies, you want to devise written discharge instructions for this population to help them or their families participate in the rehabilitation program after leaving the hospital. Discuss the factors you would consider in formulating these instructions. Then write the discharge instruction sheet according to the guidelines given in the text.

8. Review and discuss the principles for incorporating illustrations into written health care materials. Then examine your agency's client education leaflets, fact sheets, or booklets, as well as commercially prepared materials. How well do the illustrations in each group meet the criteria given in the text for effective illustrations?

9. Secure a patient package insert (PPI) for an oral contraceptive or for an estrogenic substance. Assess its readability, format, and overall appeal. Then, using the PPI and other pharmaceutical reference books, write a one-page informational/instructional fact sheet of your own about the drug for the client. Try to keep the readability level between the eighth and the tenth grades. Use diagrams or illustrations if appropriate to the material. To see how well you have communicated, test your client education tool on a sample population and on other health professionals.

10. The contracting process between nurse and client is often referred to as *contingency contracting.* Investigate the use of this term and report on your findings to the class.

11. Consider the following fact situation:

Janice Klein is the primary nurse assigned to Mrs. Claudia Jimenez, a gravida III, para O, 24-year-old Hispanic woman who is making her first visit to the city's high-risk antepartal clinic. Claudia has many chronic health problems, including juvenile-onset diabetes mellitus, essential hypertension, and severe allergies to milk and milk products. Claudia dislikes health care facilities, but because she very much wants to carry a healthy baby to term, she decides to make and keep an appointment with the clinic staff. In fact, Claudia has fears of losing another baby.

At the initial interview, Claudia tells Janice that she thought she would come "just once to see how I like this place." But it is evident to Janice that Claudia may not follow through with regular return appointments.

After Janice reviews Claudia's nursing and medical histories forwarded from the neighborhood family health clinic, she decides to suggest a nurse-client contract to Claudia as a means of encouraging her consistent return visits.

Sit in for Janice and draw up a progressive series of five or six contracts between client and nurse. Be sure to clarify the long- and short-term goals, the target dates, and the reinforcers that will help Claudia return to the high-risk clinic for careful antepartal assessment. Discuss factors in the contract that will enhance Claudia's compliance as well as those factors that will inhibit it.

REFERENCES

1. Kathleen L. Hoffland and others, "Patient Education—Developing Written Materials," *The PA Journal,* 8 (Fall 1978), 149.
2. Hoffland and others, pp. 149–162.
3. Jo-Ann Townsend, "The Unmarried, Pregnant Adolescent's Use of Educational Literature," *Nursing Outlook,* 15 (August 1967), 50.
4. John W. Scanlon, "Do Parents Need to Know More About Innocent Murmurs?" *Clinical Pediatrics,* 10 (January 1971), 24.
5. Joint Task Force for the American Diabetes Association and the American Association of Diabetes Educators, *Guidelines for Education of Patients with Diabetes Mellitus,* drafted Spring 1979.
6. Marjorie M. Crow and others, "True to Life: A Relevant Approach to Patient Education," *American Journal of Public Health,* 62 (October 1972), 1328.
7. Crow and others, p. 1330.
8. Edmund Brunner and others, *An Overview of Adult Education Research* (Washington, DC: Adult Education Association, 1959), p. 148.
9. Robert Gunning, *The Technique of Clear Writing,* 2d ed. (New York: McGraw-Hill, 1968), p. 190.

10. Mary F. Bucklin Mohammed, "Patients' Understanding of Written Health Information," *Nursing Research,* 13 (Spring 1964), 107.

11. Leonard G. Doak and Cecilia C. Doak, "Diabetes Education for Adults With Low Literacy Skills," *The Diabetes Educator,* (Winter 1978–1979), p. 16.

12. Willis A. Wingert and others, "Why Johnny's Parents Don't Read," *Clinical Pediatrics,* 8 (November 1969), 659.

13. Rudolf Flesch, *The Art of Readable Writing,* 2d ed. (New York: Harper & Row, 1974), pp. 157–158.

14. Richard R. Lanese and Randolph S. Thrush, "Measuring Readability of Health Education Literature," *Journal of the American Dietetic Association,* 42 (March 1963), 214.

15. Gunning, pp. 283–301.

16. Randolph S. Thrush and Richard R. Lanese, "The Use of Printed Material in Diabetes Education," *Diabetes,* 11 (March–April 1962), 133.

17. Thrush and Lanese, p. 136.

18. Robert Gunning, "The Fog Index After Twenty Years," in *Readings in Business Communication,* ed. Robert D. Gieselman (Champaign, IL: Stipes, 1978), p. 89.

19. Flesch, pp. 247–251.

20. Gunning, *The Technique of Clear Writing,* p. 38.

21. Gunning, *The Technique of Clear Writing,* p. 40.

22. G. Harry McLaughlin, "SMOG Grading—A New Readability Formula," *Journal of Reading,* 12 (May 1969), 640.

23. McLaughlin, p. 639.

24. Brunner and others, p. 151.

25. Florence S. Downs and Virginia Fernbach, "Experimental Evaluation of a Prenatal Leaflet Series," *Nursing Research,* 22 (November–December 1973), 505.

26. Downs and Fernbach, p. 505.

27. Ivan Barry Pless and Betty Satterwhite, "Health Education Literature for Parents of Handicapped Children," *American Journal of Diseases of Children,* 122 (September 1971), 210.

28. Scanlon, p. 24.

29. Kenneth W. Houp and Thomas E. Pearsall, *Reporting Technical Information,* 4th ed. (Encino, CA: Glencoe, 1980), p. 72.

30. Steven E. Pauley, *Technical Report Writing Today,* 2d ed. (Boston: Houghton Mifflin, 1979), pp. 125–138.

31. Sylvia L. Burkey, "An Audit Outcome: Home Going Instructions," *Supervisor Nurse,* 10 (May 1979), 36–43.

32. Burkey, p. 36.

33. Louis A. Morris and Jerome A. Halperin, "Effects of Written Drug Information on Patient Knowledge and Compliance: A Literature Review," *American Journal of Public Health,* 69 (January 1979), 51.

34. Dorothy L. Smith, *Medication Guide for Patient Counseling* (Philadelphia: Lea & Febiger, 1977), p. 21.

35. Louis A. Morris, "A Sampler of Printed Patient Oriented Prescription Drug Materials," *Drug Intelligence and Clinical Pharmacy,* 12 (March 1978), 163–164.

36. Constance Mary Clark and Elizabeth Walck Bayley, "Evaluation of the Use of Programmed Instruction for Patients Maintained on Warfarin Therapy," *American Journal of Public Health,* 62 (August 1972), 1135–1139.

37. Harriet Benson and others, "Patient Education and Intrauterine Contraception: A Study of Two Package Inserts," *American Journal of Public Health,* 67 (May 1977), 447.

38. Morris and Halperin, p. 50.

39. Evalee Keck Leeper, "Writing a Helping Hand: The Art and Technique," in *Patient and Family Education: Tools, Techniques, and Theory,* eds. Rose-Marie Duda McCormick and Tamar Gilson-Parkevich (New York: Wiley, 1979), p. 85.

40. Mary-Eve Zangari and Patricia Duffy, "Contracting With Patients in Day-to-Day Practice," *American Journal of Nursing,* 80 (March 1980), 451–452.

41. Patricia Angvik Herje, "Hows and Whys of Patient Contracting," *Nurse Educator,* 5 (January–February 1980), 30.

42. Susan Boehm Steckel and Mary Ann Swain, "Contracting With Patients to Improve Compliance," *Hospitals,* 51 (Dec. 1, 1977), 84.

43. Karyl K. Blair, "It's the Patient's Problem—and Decision," *Nursing Outlook,* 19 (September 1971), 589.

44. Herje, p. 31.

45. William J. DeRisi and George Butz, *Writing Behavioral Contracts: A Case Simulation Practice Manual* (Champaign, IL: Research Press, 1975), p. 5.

46. Rosemary Y. Wang and Joellen Watson, "Contracting for Weight Reduction—Making the Sacrifices Worthwhile," *The American Journal of Maternal Child Nursing,* 3 (January–February 1978), 46–49.

47. Steckel and Swain, p. 82.

48. Herje, p. 32.

49. Wang and Watson, p. 48.

50. DeRisi and Butz, p. 43.

51. DeRisi and Butz, p. 43.

52. Herje, p. 33.

FURTHER READING

Deberry, Pauline, and others. "Teaching Cardiac Patients to Manage Medications." *American Journal of Nursing,* 75 (December 1975), 2191–2193.

Fry, Edward. "A Readability Formula That Saves Time." *Journal of Reading,* 11 (April 1968), 513–516, 575–578.

Misik, Irene M. "Dr. Evans, Obsessed With Food, Was Starving Himself." *Nursing80,* 10 (March 1980), 54–56.

Morris, Louis A., and others. "A Survey of the Effects of Oral Contraceptive Patient Information." *Journal of the American Medical Association,* 238 (Dec. 5, 1977), 2504–2508.

Sanson-Fisher, Robert, and Kim Stotter. "Essential Steps in Designing a Successful Contract." *Child Welfare,* 56 (April 1977), 239–248.

Steckel, Susan Boehm. "Contracting With Patient-Selected Reinforcers." *American Journal of Nursing,* 80 (September 1980), 1596–1599.

CHAPTER IV

Documenting Within the Health Care System

Objectives

After studying this chapter, you will be able to

1. Explain the link between committees and agendas and minutes.
2. Differentiate among five types of committees.
3. Write a well-developed agenda for a committee meeting.
4. Record the minutes of a meeting.
5. Distinguish between procedures and policies.
6. Discuss the purposes of written procedures and the procedure manual.
7. State characteristics of the well-written procedure.
8. Analyze and critique procedures in agencies' procedure manuals.
9. Write a procedure according to the format suggested in this chapter.
10. Discuss the characteristics of written reports as they apply to incident reports and memos.
11. Define the term *incident.*
12. Discuss the most common types of reportable incidents and the factors to document when reporting them.
13. Discuss the importance of language in the incident report.
14. Write an incident report according to the general principles of incident report documentation.
15. Discuss the purposes of memos.
16. Write a brief informational memo.

In order to work successfully within a health care setting, the professional nurse must be aware of the formal lines of communication that govern the organization. Knowledge of the communication network enables the nurse to cope with the setting by devising appropriate, organizationally sanctioned means of enhancing and expediting nursing practice and the delivery of client care.

Generally expected to follow organizational lines, formal communication networks use several media to convey messages. Although the speech mode always remains important, formal networks depend on various types of written messages to systematically reach the often large number of people involved. Formal communication networks should be dynamic and free from known barriers that will hinder the flow of communication. The organizational chart is an important tool for helping the professional understand the actual flow of communication within the agency by delineating the placement of departments and positions in relation to one another.

Not only must the organization's formal communication system flow downward from top administration and management, but it must also flow upward and laterally. Although downward communication in the form of information, directives, policies, and procedures from the administrative staff is important for communicating clearly goals and means to all employees, the upward flow of communication is essential for the healthy dynamism of the system. Staff nurses who participate in committees, who help write and revise procedures, and who write periodic reports are contributing to the upward (and the lateral) flow of communication within the system.

This chapter deals with strategies for helping the professional nurse communicate effectively by appropriately using the documentation tools of the formal communication system. These tools are committees, agendas, and minutes; procedures and procedure manuals; incident reports; and memos.

COMMITTEES, AGENDAS, AND MINUTES

As a professional nurse, you may become involved in serving on a variety of committees. Although many people make light of the committee, believing that it represents the bureaucratic structure at its lowest level of efficiency, committees can be—and are—useful for achieving a variety of goals in many health care agencies.

Committees

Simply described, a committee is a group of people with a specific purpose who function collectively to attain a common goal. In other words, committees provide a means to get work done. However, committees do not sucessfully accomplish some types of work. They should not, for instance, be used to make day-to-day operating decisions that could be taken care of by an effective manager. Nor are they useful for highly complex problems that only one person should research or investigate.

According to Professor Signe S. Cooper, the basic premise underlying committees and committee work is that "problems are solved more satisfactorily and certain tasks are done more effectively by pooling the abilities, resources, interests, and experiences of several persons."[1] Thus, committees are able to make use of their diversity of membership to help identify problems, contribute ideas, clarify thinking, and develop viable solutions. Committees are especially useful—and, indeed, almost a prerequisite—for implementing major policy changes dealing with sensitive issues and for implementing successful long-range plans. And those persons who serve on a committee are more likely to support and carry out plans they helped to devise.

Basically, there are five types of committees in which nurses in health care facilities may actively participate. First, standing committees, such as the infection control committee or the nursing audit committee, traditionally deal with recurring problems or issues in the agency. Usually, standing committees have a permanent place in the agency's hierarchy through the nursing department's bylaws or the administrative bylaws. In contrast to permanent or standing committees, ad hoc ("for this case only") committees or task forces are usually set up for one specific task or purpose. Once the work is accomplished, the committee is dissolved. Cooper suggests that the difference between an ad hoc committee and a task force is nothing more than a "semantic distinction,"[2] with the term *task force* perhaps conveying the message that it is dealing with a more serious problem.

Third, multidisciplinary committees (which may be either standing or ad hoc) focus on problems or issues affecting more than one department or division. Serving on these committees with representatives from two to five different departments (such as Dietary, Administration, Pharmacy, and Physical Therapy) gives professional nurses an opportunity to represent nursing's interests as well as to broaden their knowledge about interdepartmental concerns.

Fourth, advisory committees offer counsel to a standing committee, to a department (such as staff development), or to an individual (such as the director of staff development). Finally, the fifth type of committee is one that Dr. Barbara J. Stevens views as being based on position in the organization or job function.[3] Examples of this type would be the medical head nurse committee or the clinical supervisors conference group.

Two written tools—the agenda and the minutes—help the committee realize its objectives and attain its goals.

Agendas

The agenda, that is, the committee's order of business, is usually based on the chairperson's perceptions of the committee's priorities or on the consensus of what the committee has previously identified as its priorities. The chairperson can also request committee members to suggest by a certain date items to be included on the agenda. Essentially, the purpose of the agenda is to motivate committee members to accomplish certain tasks within a reasonable time.

Because a well-formulated agenda can be written in outline form, it may be one of the easiest communications to prepare (Exhibit 4.1). Each item of business may be given an approximate time limit, to help the

Exhibit 4.1. Agenda.

ADULT NURSE PRACTITIONER COMMITTEE MEETING

APRIL 10, 1981, 7:30 AM, FIRST FLOOR CONFERENCE ROOM

1. Call to order—M. Jasco, R.N.
2. Roll call
3. Review of minutes from March 13
4. Announcements
5. Old business
   5.1 Job description
   5.2 Request for services
6. New business
   6.1 Applications for September class
   6.2 History and physical dictation
7. Adjournment

---

chairperson keep control of the meeting as well as keep it on target. Even though the agenda has a specific timetable, it should be somewhat flexible so that if a topic requires more time than originally anticipated, the time slot for another topic can be readjusted.

The agenda should not be unduly long. The chairperson must carefully estimate the time requirements of each order of business to determine whether the items on the agenda can all realistically fit into the 1-hour or 2-hour meeting. When meetings last over 2 hours, they are probably not time-effective. People become tired of sitting and often make unwise decisions, just to end an overlong session.

Most importantly, the items on the agenda should be organized in order of relative priority so that participants do not encounter the most crucial issues at the conclusion of the meeting. When issues are not arranged according to priority, they should at least be arranged so that the first item leads naturally into the second, and the second leads naturally into the third, and so on.

The agenda should be formulated and distributed to committee members *several days before* the scheduled meeting. Such timing is advantageous for four reasons:

1. The agenda contains the date, time, and place of the forthcoming meeting, and so it serves as a notification and verification of the meeting.
2. Participants can prepare by knowing in advance what is to be discussed. Members are able to formulate their positions, review any reports, articles, or printed information included with the agenda, and

prepare a list of questions to assist the group in considering all aspects of the items listed.

3. In certain cases, participants may feel the need to poll others informally about the group's stand on vital issues on the agenda.
4. Participants are thus reminded to bring along materials, equipment, or the results of formal or informal surveys, to facilitate the committee's work.

The actual format of the agenda may vary according to the agency, the nature of the committee, and the issues or problems to be dealt with. We recommend that professional nurses who serve on committees become acquainted with *Robert's Rules of Order* to help them with the rudiments of parliamentary procedure. This book can supply a starting point when you have to prepare an agenda. Most likely, however, you will need to revise the order and plan the agenda to reflect the needs of the committee and the purpose of the meeting.

One possible agenda format is as follows:

- Call to order
- Roll call
- Review of minutes from previous meeting
- Announcements
- Subcommittee reports
- Old business
- New business
- Adjournment

Minutes

Minutes are the official record of the committee's proceedings. They should be available to participants *well before* the next meeting so that all can see the record of the committee's proceedings (Exhibit 4.2). In some instances, one person is appointed as the recorder for a given number of consecutive meetings. On the other hand, many committees rotate the recording duty with each meeting, to enable all to share the responsibility of taking the minutes. Moreover, rotating this duty prevents the same member from always being less than a fully active participant because he or she must focus on writing during the meetings.

Minutes have several purposes—to summarize and record discussion, to record decisions, to note progress toward goals and objectives, and to

Exhibit 4.2. Minutes.

ADULT NURSE PRACTITIONER COMMITTEE
MINUTES OF THE APRIL 10 MEETING

The regular meeting of the Adult Nurse Practitioner Committee was called to order at 7:30 AM on Thursday, April 10, 1981, in the first floor conference room. M. Jasco, R.N., presided.

PRESENT: L. Browning, M.D., V. Claystreet, R.N., M. Stein, M.D., S. Wittenhouse, R.N., B. Yarborough, R.N.

ABSENT: J. Krull, R.N.

MINUTES: The minutes of the March 13 meeting were reviewed and approved.

ANNOUNCEMENTS: S. Wittenhouse has submitted her letter of resignation, effective June 30, due to moving out of state.

JOB DESCRIPTION: B. Yarborough distributed the revised draft of the Nurse Practitioner Job Description. The committee unanimously approved the revisions.

REQUEST FOR SERVICES: V. Claystreet distributed the form that physicians will sign when they request the services of a nurse practitioner. The form states that physicians will cosign the practitioner's histories and physical assessments as well as all standing orders within 24 hours. The committee unanimously approved the form, and M. Stein will present it to Executive Council for approval on April 15.

NEXT PRACTITIONER CLASS: All R.N.s who meet the preestablished criteria are eligible to apply for the September class. M. Jasco will send out a memo tomorrow to all nursing divisions informing them that applications for the next class will be available in the education office from April 15 to April 30. The committee will review the applications during its regularly scheduled May meeting.

HISTORY AND PHYSICAL DICTATION: Nurse practitioner students have not been able to obtain access to the dictating equipment in Medical Records. L. Browning and M. Jasco will set up an appointment with A. Griffith to investigate what routes can be taken so that nurse practitioners may dictate.

NEXT MEETING: The next meeting will be held on May 2, 1981, at 8 AM in the fifth floor conference room.

ADJOURNMENT: The meeting was adjourned at 8:45 AM.

K. Singleton, R.N.

record actions and the delegation of assignments. They can quickly bring missing members up to date on the activities and decisions of the previous meeting. They provide new members with a kind of historical perspective on the committee's goals, activities, and past successes and failures. They also ease the writing of progress reports or an annual report for the clinical director or administrator.

In general, minutes do not have to be excessively detailed. But if the committee should want them to be very complete, taping a session may be more effective than taking written notes. Transcribing a tape, however, especially for a 2-hour meeting, can prove a time-consuming and tedious chore. It might be better, then, to have a clerk typist or a secretary with dictation skills record a meeting for which very complete minutes are required. Later, the official recorder could help the secretary determine the wording and the content of the proceedings.

Some agencies use a specific, semistructured format to record the proceedings of a committee or conference. If your agency does not specify a format, you can follow the agenda format as an aid in organizing the minutes. We recommend the following format:

- Name of committee
- Date, time, and place
- Attendance—present, absent, excused
- Review of minutes of last meeting
- Announcements
- Progress reports or officer reports
- Old business—motions, decisions, actions
- New business—motions, decisions, actions
- Next meeting date, time, and place
- Adjournment time
- Recorder's signature and typed name

Today's professional nurse needs to know not only *the how* but also *the why* behind committees, agendas, and minutes.

PROCEDURES AND PROCEDURE MANUALS

Nurses at many agencies often become involved in formulating, writing, revising, and evaluating various types of procedures, including those related to standards of nursing practice and those related to the general operation of the nursing department. Nurses may be formally appointed to the agency's procedure committee, or they may be asked, because of their clinical knowledge or expertise, to participate as ad hoc members to write, revise, or evaluate selected procedures. Even though several fine procedure references (such as Dison's *Clinical Nursing Techniques,* Brunner and Suddarth's *Lippincott Manual of Nursing Practice,* and King's *Illustrated Manual of Nursing Techniques*) have been published in the past few years, most agencies continue to maintain their own written procedures and procedure manuals. But as Lyla Niederbaumer points out, because the procedure book is a time-consuming and expensive manual to write and produce, it behooves nurses who participate in writing procedures to do so in the most effective way.[4]

As specific, concrete guides to action, procedures delineate the chronological or sequential order in which the steps of the action or process are to be performed. Agency procedures are usually generated from two sources: (1) general nursing practice principles and (2) agency policies on nursing practice or the general operation of Nursing Service.

The first type of nursing procedures—those based on nursing practice principles—may be viewed as action vehicles or operational tools that the nurse uses to implement client-centered nursing care. Procedures are guidelines to responsible nursing actions, based on well-established nursing principles and principles from the biological and social sciences.

The second type of procedures will originate from the agency's operational policies. Now, policies have been variously defined as rules "for human conduct formulated with a particular intention in mind,"[5] as guidelines for governing "individual managers in their decision-making,"[6] and as guidelines "for decisions regarding actions."[7] Thus, policies provide general direction in decision making so that action can be taken within the framework of the organization's beliefs and principles. A policy, however, cannot substitute for the detailed procedure by which it is to be implemented. In effect, then, procedures are the mechanisms or tools to standardize the implementation of agency policies or nursing principles.

There are several reasons for agencies to compile their own manuals of procedures rather than to rely completely on the available procedure references. Agency procedure manuals often supply cross-references to their associated policies, protocols, and standards—a feature that would be missing in general procedure references. And many nursing procedures must be adapted to become congruent with agency policies.

Whether an agency relies on a general reference for many of its procedures or on its own manual, written procedures are important for the following five reasons:

1. They standardize operational mechanisms or steps in a complex process. This aspect is especially valuable since many facilities employ all levels of personnel coming from a variety of educational and experiential backgrounds.
2. They help ensure uniformity of performance, thus promoting the consistency of client care. For example, if an agency's urine testing procedure for diabetic clients is to test only second-voided specimens obtained 20 to 30 minutes after the first voiding, it is crucial that this procedure be clearly written in the manual, to help maintain a consistent approach.
3. They provide a readily available, current reference to refamiliarize nurses with complex procedures infrequently performed. Nurses on

the neuroorthopedic unit may rarely participate in preparing a client for a thoracentesis. But when they have to, they have access to the agency's procedure manual to bring them up to date on the equipment they must gather, their role in preparing and instructing the client, and their role in assisting the physician.

4. They provide a standard to help in the evaluation of the delivery of nursing care. The standard that the procedure conveys is especially valuable when nonprofessional personnel are involved in the delivery or performance of selected nursing procedures.

5. They provide standardized guidelines and/or instructions for the use of equipment. Since many pieces of equipment are costly, it is essential that all personnel know how to operate them or use them safely and efficiently. Good procedures tell personnel how the equipment can be obtained, how to operate it safely, how to clean it before returning it to the central dispensing area, and the precautions needed in its use with clients in isolation.

Procedure Manual Content and Organization

The content and organization of the procedure manual depend on the audience for whom the manual is intended. If all levels of nursing personnel—from aide and orderly to clinical supervisor—use the book, then it seems likely that all procedures performed at the agency should be included. Niederbaumer argues, however, that because most aides, orderlies, and nursing assistants have had some type of "pre-service"[8] training classes or orientation, agency manuals need not include such basic procedures as making beds or feeding clients. Procedures that merely detail one's initial nursing instruction could be safely omitted from the agency's procedure book as long as they are included in the facility's training manual.

The procedure manual is usually organized into a large loose-leaf notebook so that obsolete, new, and revised procedures may be readily added or deleted. Copies are produced in sufficient quantities so that every nursing unit has one. Procedures should be arranged alphabetically, with a carefully devised cross-reference system, so that procedures that could be filed under more than one category can be easily located.

Another organizational system that has proved very workable consists of a revolving card file.[9] The size of the cards (5" × 8") helps keep the procedures succinct. And since the plastic-protected cards can be easily removed from the file, nurses can take the appropriate card or cards with them as they prepare for an unfamiliar or complex procedure.

Procedure Format

There are many formats in which meaningful procedures can be written. As long as the format adequately conveys what the person must do to carry out the procedure effectively, logically, and safely, the format need not cause great concern. Selecting a good procedure format helps you work more efficiently by supplying structure and guidelines, just as using an appropriate format would prove helpful in other writing situations.

Traditional procedure formats have included such heading categories as purpose, equipment, procedure, and charting.[10] Margaret L. Wright suggests using a combined definition and purpose statement, followed by a list of general instructions, required materials, and the steps needed to complete the job.[11] Sharon Riutta describes a format that reflects one agency's belief that procedures, just like the delivery of care, should reflect client-centered care and not simply the performance of tasks. Since her agency views the procedure as an integral part of the plan of care, the selected format incorporates elements of the nursing process. Heading categories include, therefore, five elements: objective, preparation and teaching, implementation, documentation, and additional information.[12]

We recommend a format that consists of these nine elements:

1. Procedure title
2. Definition
3. Purpose
4. Equipment
5. Client preparation
6. Related information
7. Procedure steps
8. Documentation
9. Follow-up care

Exhibit 4.3 illustrates the nine elements in action in the heparin lock procedure.

The first three elements—procedure title, definition, and purpose—identify and structure the procedure. Giving the procedure a succinct and appropriate title helps guard against incomplete indexing or cross-referencing. A good definition serves to clarify the procedure in light of agency policy. A concise phrase should be sufficient. The purpose, usually expressed with the infinitive verb form, provides the objective(s) of the procedure.

The next three elements—equipment, client preparation, and related information—make up the preparation phase. The equipment section lists supplies the nurse must gather, including the location of and means for requisitioning items not stocked on the unit. Client preparation includes the physical and emotional or psychological aspects of care, as well as the nurse's teaching duties.

Exhibit 4.3. Procedure.

HEPARIN LOCK

DEFINITION: The insertion of an indwelling needle for the use of intermittent doses of IV medication, kept patent by means of a diluted heparin solution

PURPOSE: 1. To spare the client unnecessary trauma from multiple venipunctures
2. To minimize the number of veins used for the administration of medications given intermittently
3. To allow the client greater mobility by eliminating cumbersome IV tubing, bottles, and armboards

EQUIPMENT: 1. Povidone iodine prep
2. 1 No. 19 or No. 21 intermittent infusion needle
3. 1 roll each ¼" and ½" hypoallergenic tape
4. I tb syringe
5. 100 units of sodium heparin (from a 10-cc vial of sodium heparin 1,000 units/cc)
6. 30-cc vial of sterile normal saline
7. Tourniquet
8. 1 5-cc. syringe of normal saline with a small-gauge (No. 25) needle
9. 1 package antibiotic ointment
10. Alcohol preps

CLIENT PREPARATION: 1. Explain the purpose of the heparin lock to the client, emphasizing its advantages: comfort, mobility, and fewer venipunctures.
2. Instruct the client about the medications he or she will be receiving via the heparin lock.
3. Teach the client to recognize and report signs and symptoms of infiltration: burning, redness, warmth, soreness, and pain.

RELATED INFORMATION: A diluted heparin holding solution must be instilled after the lock set is inserted and after each dose of medication, to prevent the formation of clots and fibrinous materials.

PROCEDURE STEPS

Nursing Actions	Key Points
1. Identify the client and explain the procedure.	
2. Prepare the heparin holding solution in the medication room by diluting 0.1 cc of heparin (1,000 units/cc) with 0.9 cc of normal saline.	
3. Assemble the equipment at the bedside.	
4. Wash your hands.	
5. Cleanse the proposed injection site thoroughly with povidone iodine.	Allow to dry for at least 1 minute.

169

Exhibit 4.3. (Continued)

PROCEDURE STEPS

Nursing Actions	Key Points
6. Cleanse the rubber port of the heparin lock with alcohol.	
7. Insert the 5-cc syringe of saline with a No. 25 gauge needle into the injection port.	The small-gauge needle prevents extensive punctures of the rubber diaphragm.
8. Flush the heparin lock tubing reservoir with 1 cc of saline.	Leave the needle and syringe attached to the port after flushing the reservoir with saline.
9. Apply a tourniquet 2 to 5 in (5 to 13 cm) above the proposed venipuncture site.	Select a vein large enough to allow for rapid dilution of the medication, thereby preventing venous irritation.
10. Perform the venipuncture.	
11. Release the tourniquet.	
12. Aspirate for blood return.	
13. Secure the needle with one piece of ¼″ hypoallergenic tape over the needle wings.	Be sure the tape does not touch venipuncture site.
14. Write the date, time of insertion, and nurse's initials on a piece of ½″ tape; place it over the first piece of tape.	
15. Inject 2 cc of saline to assure patency.	If the client complains of signs and symptoms of infiltration, discontinue the heparin lock and restart it aseptically at another site.
16. Apply antibiotic ointment to the insertion site; cover it with a sterile adhesive bandage.	
17. Secure the tubing with additional tape as needed.	
18. Remove the saline syringe from the injection port.	
19. Wipe the port with alcohol and insert the syringe containing diluted heparin solution.	
20. Instill 0.3 to 0.5 cc of diluted heparin solution.	The solution will clear the reservoir and keep the vein patent until the prescribed medication is administered.

DOCUMENT:
1. Date
2. Time
3. Size of heparin lock
4. Location
5. Client's reaction to the procedure

Exhibit 4.3. (Continued)

FOLLOW-UP CARE:	1. Inspect the insertion site a minimum of twice per shift for signs and symptoms of infiltration. 2. Follow up the client's understanding of reporting signs and symptoms of infiltration to the nurse. 3. Change the dressing daily. See procedure: "Intravenous Infusions: Daily Dressing Change."

The actual steps of the procedure constitute the performance phase of the process. Frequently, these steps are presented in a two-column format, with one column labeled "Nursing Actions" and the other labeled "Key Points." Nursing actions are the sequential steps in the process; key points amplify the reasoning behind the steps. Such reasoning becomes especially important if the agency's procedure varies significantly from recognized standards or commonly accepted principles. It is in this procedure steps section that general policies and principles related to safety, infection control, and legalities (such as securing informed consent) are typically addressed. Nursing actions begin with specific action verbs; key points may or may not require complete sentences, for often a phrase will make the meaning clear.

Finally, the documentation and follow-up care sections tell the nurse where to chart the procedure and what measures to take (including precautions and nursing observations) to follow up the procedure.

Writing the Procedure

You should remember two fundamental points in the writing of procedures. First, procedure writing deals with a *process,* that is, a specific series of actions that bring about a specific change or result. Usually, a process involves chronological or sequential events, moving from beginning to end. And since they reflect a process, procedures tend to get written according to a relatively fixed order of events in which there is basically one correct way to arrange the steps. But there may be times when the procedure does not need to reflect the more "rigid" chronological or sequential fixed order to achieve the desired results. In this case, the procedure writer can use a more flexible order of choice, based perhaps on a logical way of organizing the procedure according to what those who routinely perform the procedure have identified as efficient, logical, or helpful.

Second, for the procedure to communicate effectively the process and for the process to be performed well, you should write understandable instructions. Characteristics of effective instructions include

- An uncluttered, straightforward style
- Specific action verbs
- The imperative mood
- Short sentences, usually in the range of 10 to 20 words
- A precise, meaningful vocabulary
- Strategically placed "warnings" or "cautions"
- Carefully prepared diagrams or illustrations, placed as close as possible to the instruction

When the procedure contains a complex process, you can divide it into its major phases or steps and then write the instructions for each phase in sequence or according to a logical order of choice. Dividing the process into more easily manageable content will make writing the procedure easier.

As you might expect, there are some other things to keep in mind when you write, revise, or review procedures. Clearly, you should determine the relationship between agency policy and procedure. You recall that procedures are the "how to" or the operational guidelines to put policies into action. Thus, unless you know what the agency's policy is concerning the registered nurse's role in drawing arterial blood gases, you will not be able to write a very effective procedure in that instance.

Furthermore, if you must write a completely new procedure for something that has never been performed before by nurses at the facility, you can use selected references for appropriate background information. Current textbooks of medical-surgical nursing, procedure references, journal articles, package inserts, and manufacturers' instructions provide excellent sources for the principles and mechanics of carrying out a procedure. In fact, it is wise to consult current sources about *any* procedure *before* reviewing or revising that procedure. Occasionally, because the procedure writer has neglected to check recent literature, routinely performed procedures remain unchanged for several years, despite new information or research on the principles or policies upon which they are based.

Whether procedures are being written for the first time or routinely reviewed and revised, it is also advisable to ask those personnel who carry out the procedure for their suggestions. "People will carry the procedure out more conscientiously if they feel they have a stake in it,"[13] maintains nursing consultant Lillian S. Brunner. And whether you review a procedure or you ask someone else with clinical expertise to review it, be sure you actually go through the performance steps to catch errors in sequence or logic, omissions of essential steps, and ways to delete or combine steps.

Finally, to evaluate your effectiveness in writing procedures, ask yourself the following questions:

1. Have I based my procedure on the agency's written policy? Does the procedure successfully put the policy into action?
2. Have I based the procedure on sound, up-to-date principles from the nursing literature if no written agency policy applies to the procedure?
3. Does the procedure fulfill its purpose(s)?
4. Have I written the procedure steps clearly and logically?
5. Have I used appropriate instructional language for the procedure steps—action verbs, imperative mood, short sentences, and precise vocabulary?
6. If I have used illustrations, are they clear? Do they augment the written instructions? Are they appropriate to the steps they illustrate?
7. Have I incorporated into the procedure policies or principles related to safety, infection control, and legal concerns?
8. Have I shown the procedure to nurses with clinical expertise and asked for their suggestions? Have I incorporated their revisions?
9. Have I written the procedure so that a new employee (or someone who has not done this procedure before) can perform it satisfactorily after reading just one time what I have written?

INCIDENT REPORTS

Nurses in all areas of practice prepare reports. Nurses at acute care agencies report formally through oral and written channels on clients' progress or change of status during a specific time period, usually 8 hours. They often complete written supervisors' reports, maintenance or safety reports, and evaluations of products, employees, or mechanical or informational systems. Routinely, they report diabetic reactions, results of transfusions, and suspected drug reactions. Public health nurses write progress reports on their clients for physicians and other health care agencies. School health nurses must report children's deviations from the normal patterns of growth and development. And nurses at extended care facilities must write a full report on their clients' biopsychosocial status every month.

The reports that nurses make may vary considerably according to degree of formality, mode of transmission, and length. In general, a report is an oral or written message designed to convey information, identify problems, or present solutions. Reports may be classified according to function, length, formality, and frequency of issue, just to name a few ways. Reports classified by function include informational reports and analytical reports. Informational reports simply present data, with no attempt to analyze or interpret the meaning of the data or to make any recommendations for action. Analytical reports, however, provide information as well as analysis, interpretation, or recommendations.

One very important and frequently written type of report in health care facilities is the incident report. Analytical by nature, most incident reports request observable, factual data, as well as ask the writer to analyze the events that may have led up to, precipitated, or contributed to the incident. We may define an incident as an unusual occurrence, that is, an unexpected happening that is not consistent with the routine operation of the agency or the routine care of a particular client. An incident may cause injury or have the potential to cause harm or injury to a client, visitor, or employee. Misplaced, lost, and damaged items belonging to either client or visitor are included. Health care facilities need a viable incident reporting mechanism to enable them to comply with government regulations for promptly reporting employee accidents and injuries. They also use the incident report to document any accidents or unusual happenings for their insurance companies or lawyers in the event that suit is brought against the agency.

Incident reports are internal administrative documents that alert top management that something unusual has happened. All incidents must be recorded and reported, whether or not there is apparent harm or damage. As Shannon E. Perry aptly points out, "Although the injury may not appear serious . . . the incident form should be filled out. Injuries can surface later, and it is important to have written documentation of the event. . . ."[14] Although the literature on incident reports reflects some debate about whether a copy of an incident report belongs in the client's record, those agencies with active risk management committees tend to view the report as a confidential document that should be seen only by the administration, its insurance company, or its attorneys. Some agencies include a copy of the incident report in the chart after the client is discharged, but it does not become a permanent part of his or her record.

During the early 1970s, when insurance and malpractice premiums rose dramatically, many health care facilities became active participants in risk management in order to identify those risks, problems, and safety concerns that could reduce the agency's effectiveness in providing a generally risk-free environment. Because the first step in the risk management process is identifying potential or actual risks, the incident report is an essential tool for helping agency administrators, safety committees, and risk management coordinators pinpoint and analyze problems.

Purposes of the Incident Report

As an integral part of the risk management program, the incident report has several purposes. First, it notifies the administration, insurance carriers, and legal counsel that an unusual occurrence has taken place— perhaps one that could lead to litigation against the agency. Prompt communication of the details of the unusual occurrence may help the administrative staff provide immediate follow-up action to eliminate or minimize the impact of the incident. Because the incident report documents the details of the event while they are still fresh in the observer's memory, the report is an excellent means of helping to assess the agency's liability in the event of a lawsuit. If allegations are made, a well-documented incident report can help the agency refute the charges by demonstrating that reasonable precautions were taken to protect the client from injury or loss.

Over a period of time, moreover, the incident report helps in developing a statistical basis for summarizing data that may not be significant individually but that may reveal a pattern of accidents when examined altogether. Or the reports may reveal a close correlation between specific data (age, sex, time of day, location, etc.) and a certain type of incident.

Education is another purpose of the incident report. Writing the report demands that employees scrutinize the possible relationships between unsafe practices and negative client or employee outcomes. Based on the trends or patterns identified in the reported data, staff development programs can be planned to refamiliarize personnel with their responsibilities for safe client care and to minimize those high-risk incidents.

Perhaps what is most important for staff to realize, however, is that the purpose of the report is *not* to criticize or discipline; rather, it is to improve care and/or identify standards for safe client care.

Categories of Reportable Incidents

Even though our definition of the term *incident* should indicate fairly well what you should be reporting, it may be helpful to survey the most common categories of reportable incidents and the factors to document when reporting them. Falls, medication or treatment errors, patient-inherent occurrences, loss of personal effects, and defective equipment or an unsafe environment are the five categories we will review.

Falls account for 75% of the incidents reported on the clinical units, according to the data of researcher Frances H. Lynn.[15] Frequently, clients fall while ambulating, but they may also fall while moving from wheelchair to bed, while showering, while getting in or out of the tub, and while getting out of bed. They may trip over tubing, bump into furniture, or slip on wet floors. Elderly hospitalized clients are even more susceptible to falls, as a recent *American Journal of Nursing* article entitled "Why the Elderly Fall" explains so well.[16]

When reporting a fall from bed, you should state the height of the bed as well as whether the client was restrained and whether both siderails were up. In documenting *all* falls, be sure to report the floor's condition (wet or dry), the presence of equipment around the bed or the area where the client was ambulating, the use of self-help devices (canes, walkers, crutches), and any observable physiological responses (vital signs, level of consciousness, location and appearance of cuts, bruises, or lacerations). If the client complains of pain, quote the person's exact words in the report. You should also include any relevant environmental details that may have contributed to the fall.

Another type of incident involves medication or treatment errors. Some agencies use a separate form to report medication errors, but the basic concept of reporting remains the same as for other incidents. In "The Classification of Medication Errors," Joanna L. Apple suggests that errors in procedure account for the largest percentage of medication errors.[17] Procedural mistakes include making a transcription error, misreading the medication card, failing to use the medication card, omitting a prescribed dose, or administering the wrong medicine. In addition, medication errors can occur through dosage (miscalculating or measuring incorrectly) or route (e.g., administering a medication intramuscularly when it should have been given orally).

When reporting medication or treatment incidents, you will see the need for not only objective information or data but also interpretation or analysis of the problem. At this point, the analytical function of report writing enters the picture. Some analysis of the reason for an error can help nursing staff, the safety committee, nursing administration, and the risk management coordinator identify and eliminate conditions that contribute to errors. To explain the nature of a medication incident, for example, the nurse may write: "Aldoril-25 given at 3 PM instead of Aldomet 250 mg." The causative agent should be identified, whether it is a transcription error, an unclear medicine card, or a mislabeled medication. If the pharmacy contributed to the error by misreading the physician's order and sending the incorrect medication to the unit, this should also be documented. In reporting medication or treatment errors, you should specify the corrective action taken to prevent the error from occurring again or to safeguard the client's status after the incident. Some corrective actions might be returning the medication to the pharmacy for relabeling or scheduling a unit inservice program. If the incident is serious, corrective action may be governed by the physician's therapeutic regimen, such as monitoring vital signs and obtaining immediate blood work or diagnostic tests.

Patient-inherent occurrences compose the third category of reportable incidents. The term *patient-inherent* refers to mishaps, other than falls, that are caused by clients themselves. Lynn cites "self-inflicted cuts, burns from hot fluids, collisions, ingestion or incorporation of foreign substances, self-mutilation, setting fires, or pinching fingers in drawers or doors"[18] as some examples. In suspected patient-inherent incidents, you should document what you have seen as objectively as possible. If a staff member did not see the incident occur, it is helpful to note the name of the client's roommate or visitor who witnessed the incident.

Fourth, incidents involving the loss of clothing, money, dentures, glasses, and various prostheses must be reported as soon as they are noticed. Many agencies supply personal property lists for itemizing the clients' effects when they are admitted. In this way, staff members can know what clients brought with them so that all items can be accounted for when they leave. If such a list is used, clients and their families should be instructed to tell the nursing staff when they bring additional items to the agency and when they send them home before discharge. A careful inventory of personal property helps decrease the risk of loss or theft. Some agencies request that clients send large sums of money or other valuables to the vault for safekeeping; some request that clients not bring such items with them in the first place.

When reporting the loss or theft of personal property, nursing personnel should use the specific description of the item that the client or the family provides. The last date and time the item was seen by the staff or the family should be given. Because losing personal articles such as hearing aids or dentures may be very upsetting to a client, every effort should be made to find them at the same time that the administration is notified—orally and in writing—of the incident. The client's bed linen can be checked, and the laundry and housekeeping departments can be alerted.

The last category of client-related incidents includes defective equipment or an unsafe environment. Actually, improperly functioning equipment or less than adequate environmental conditions may *be* incidents as well as *cause* other types of incidents, most typically slips and falls. Adjustable walkers with loose screws, crutches with ill-fitting rubber tips, wheelchairs with malfunctioning brakes, loose floor tile, and burned-out light bulbs could be causative agents. In short, whether the malfunctioning equipment was an incident per se or else contributed to an incident, the circumstances surrounding the event should be clearly documented, with answers to such questions as *who, what, when, where,* and *how much.*

The following excerpt from a report describes an incident specifically and objectively:

> The client was ambulating down the north corridor with a walker and the help of Ms. Koss, nursing assistant. Ms. Koss was walking behind and 30 degrees to the left of the client, holding on to the gait belt around his waist. Suddenly, the rubber tips on the walker's right and left front legs came off, causing the client to lose his balance and be propelled forward. He did not fall; he was steadied by Ms. Koss's hold on the gait belt. Immediately afterward, the client complained of a "terrible pain" along the inner aspect of his right leg, from the groin to the proximal third of the calf.

> Ms. Koss and I inspected the floor after the client was assisted to the wheelchair. It was dry and free from loose objects and equipment.

> With his right leg extended, the client was returned to bed via the wheelchair. Dr. Paul Jones was called and will see the client within 1 half-hour. The walker and rubber tips were returned to Maintenance for evaluation and repair, along with a written explanation of what happened.

Authorship of the Incident Report

As a rule, the person who discovers the incident, particularly one involving client injuries, writes the incident report. But since the registered nurse is ultimately responsible for client care, she or he usually writes the report when the incident occurs on the nursing unit. In some agencies, moreover, the person who discovers the incident is obligated to report first to the head nurse or nurse in charge. These two people then jointly document the event. This practice may be especially beneficial when the person who discovered the incident is an ancillary care giver who is not accustomed to documenting reports as carefully as do professional nurses. The practice of joint report writing may be unnecessary, however, on nursing units staffed with a high percentage of professional nurses.

Of course, if the incident occurs while the client is off the unit, the staff person (physical therapist or x-ray technician, for example) who discovers the incident or accompanies the client makes the report.

Format of the Incident Report

Incident report formats vary from agency to agency, according to its history of past incidents, previously identified risk factors, and the information required by the insurance carrier. Some facilities have separate forms for clients, visitors, and employees. Other agencies use one form for clients, visitors, and volunteers (Exhibit 4.4) but a different one for employees. In some agencies, nursing personnel use a special form for documenting medication errors, but elsewhere they may report them on the standard incident report form.

Information in the incident report can be categorized into three separate areas: (1) baseline data, (2) description of the incident and resulting actions taken, and (3) physician's statement.

Baseline data are gathered for both background and statistical purposes. They assist the risk management coordinator or the administrator in more easily classifying incidents according to their associated risk factors and in gaining a better understanding of the environment in which they occurred. You can expeditiously gather the data by stamping the form with the client's addressograph plate and by entering the appropriate information, from date, time, and location to position of bed, medications given before incident, type of incident, person who discovered incident, and name of report writer, among others. Again, you can get a good idea of what is included in baseline data by reviewing the incident report sheet reproduced in Exhibit 4.4.

The description of the incident and the resulting actions taken by the nurse should be carefully set forth in a clear, readable style. Since the basis of the incident report is factual information, the report writer describes the mishap in an orderly, progressive manner, exactly as the events occurred. If a member of the nursing staff did not see the incident, the writer should document the event according to what the client or witness is able to say. Whenever possible, the client's exact words should be quoted. Thus, instead of generalizing that "client seemed unsure of how she fell," it is more precise and factual to quote her directly: " 'I just felt dizzy all of a sudden, and I guess I fell. I don't remember hitting my head, but I must have. It really hurts.' "

The narrative should also contain the nurse's observations of the client (or the person involved) and the surroundings, as well as the appropriate actions taken to prevent further harm or injury from occurring. *Reportable observations* include vital signs; level of consciousness and/or emotional status; size, color, and location of bruises, cuts, or abrasions; presence and degree of draining wounds or bleeding; complaints of pain or immobility; and the condition of any involved equipment. *Reportable actions* include initiating emergency measures, calling the physician, as-

Exhibit 4.4. Incident report.

INCIDENT REPORT   Give name and address of person involved. Use imprinter for clients.

DATE OF INCIDENT _____ TIME OF INCIDENT _____
LOCATION _____
INCIDENT INVOLVED   Client _____ Visitor _____ Volunteer _____ Other _____
SEX   M _____ F _____ Age _____

IF PERSON INVOLVED WAS CLIENT   DIAGNOSIS _____
BED RAILS PRESENT?   Yes _____ No _____ Up _____ Down _____
ADJUSTABLE BED?   Yes _____ No _____ Up _____ Down _____
CLIENT'S CONDITION BEFORE INCIDENT   Normal _____ Disoriented _____ Sedated _____
Unresponsive _____ Other _____
MEDICATIONS GIVEN DURING PAST 6 HOURS _____
TYPE OF INCIDENT   Slip and Fall _____ Medication _____ Procedure _____ Loss _____
Other _____

DESCRIBE INCIDENT (include nature of harm or injury, primary causes, pertinent vital signs,
and any involved equipment)

NAMES/ADDRESSES OF WITNESSES _____

NAME OF NURSING SUPERVISOR NOTIFIED _____ TIME _____
NAME OF PHYSICIAN NOTIFIED _____ TIME _____
EXAMINATION BY PHYSICIAN   Yes _____ No _____ Refused _____
INCIDENT DISCOVERED BY _____ REPORT PREPARED BY _____
EXAMINING PHYSICIAN'S STATEMENT

SIGNATURE _____

---

sisting the client back to bed, or moving the client by stretcher or wheelchair. The client's response to emergency or immediate medical intervention should also be recorded.

In this section of the report, which describes the incident, the nurse must be especially careful to avoid vague or unclear terms and statements. If a physician is called to see the client, it is important to give his or her complete name. Statements such as "Resident notified" or "Attending physician called" should not appear, for there may be many on-call residents on the staff of a large facility or there may be more than one attending physician caring for the client. Terms such as *quite, apparently,* and *seemingly* detract from the objectivity of the report. You should document quantitative information as concretely as possible. "Several minutes" is less meaningful than "5 or 6 minutes"; "cut on forehead" is less accurate than "1.5-cm laceration above left eyebrow." In sum, the prudent nurse reviews and proofreads the description of the incident and the actions taken—*before signing*—to be certain that the report is factual, understandable, and free from ambiguous language.

The third section of the report concerns notifying the appropriate physician of the incident and then entering the exact time of your call together with the response to your call. In critical situations, it may be necessary to document being unable to reach the physician as well as the number of times you have tried to contact the physician. Later, the physician will add a statement about the client's condition or injury, order any necessary tests, and also sign the report.

In short, to write effective incident reports, you should

1. Follow the agency's policies and procedures on the prompt reporting of incidents.
2. Submit the written report to the risk management coordinator, administrator, or safety committee chairperson as soon as possible, usually within 24 hours after the incident takes place. Also, orally notify the responsible person about potentially serious incidents.
3. Use factual, concise, and unambiguous language.
4. Avoid vague terms such as *may, seems, apparently, somewhat, several,* and *few.*
5. Use appropriate anatomical landmarks and exact measurements to describe the precise location of the injury, pain, or immobility.
6. Quote the client or involved person directly, to avoid making judgmental or sometimes incorrect inferences.
7. Describe the incident using a narrative style that reflects the order or logical progression of the events leading up to the incident, the incident, and what occurred afterward.

8. Review and proofread the completed report before signing it, to be sure it is clear and accurate.

MEMOS

Memos probably have the greatest potential of all written reports for inundating the nurse working in a health care facility. One glance at your nursing unit's bulletin boards, communication book, or memo clipboard should illustrate out point. In just 1 week's time, a nursing division may receive 15 to 20 memos from *other* departments in the agency, and it may well generate the same number intradepartmentally. Yet there is no doubt that memos are a convenient means of communication when they are used properly. And sometimes they can be a marvelous vehicle for presenting routine information with an appropriately humorous twist, as the attention-getting memo in Exhibit 4.5 demonstrates. Tom Sadvary's *Fly Wars* memo takes a new look at an old problem. It also uses the direct structure (big idea, explanation, summary) and a special list for maximum clarity.

Essentially, memos are brief, informational messages, usually less than one page. Because memos are internal communications for use *within* an agency or organization, they are often informally written, sometimes even handwritten. Of course, longer or more complex memos are carefully typed. Memo format traditionally contains four headings at the top of the page after the agency's logo: Date, To, From, and Subject. The subject line should indicate the memo's content accurately and specifically. Some agencies require that memos be signed at the end as are letters, but most agencies recommend that writers simply initial each memo next to their typed name in the heading.

Memos communicate *upward* to superiors and *downward* to subordinates. They can also foster *lateral* communication between personnel of equal rank. As a nurse in a health care facility, you may receive memos directed to you personally that notify you of a meeting or of your appointment to a committee or that confirm a change of position or working hours. You may also be affected by memos sent to the nursing staff from the nursing department, from ancillary departments, and from the administrative staff.

There are several advantages to writing and sending effective memos. For example, policy statements first presented orally but then confirmed in writing clarify the policy and related directive by forcing the memo sender to plan the message carefully to avoid producing noise and subse-

bch
barberton citizens
hospital
Memo

TO: All Departments/Divisions/Nursing Units   **DATE:** August 8, 198_

FROM: Tom Sadvary, Assistant Administrator

SUBJECT: Fly Wars, Chapter 1

THE BCH FLY BRIGADE WANTS YOU!

After a series of ruthless attacks by the Barberton fly community, Barberton Citizens Hospital has declared an all-out war against these pesky and dirty critters. A fly brigade has been formed, and the following steps have been taken, using both traditional and highly sophisticated measures (this is more than a fly-by-night attempt!):

  *Purchasing two additional electronic "flowtron fly killers," which work on a black light principle and are ecologically safe. These expensive but effective anti-fly devices will be strategically placed in the Cafeteria, where the fly population is the heaviest.

  *Purchasing several "fly strips," rolled flypaper, if you will. This is primitive, but effective, and available from the Purchasing Department upon request. However, contact Infection Control (X 5435) to make sure that it's O.K. to use these devices in your area.

  *Contacting the Barberton Health Department, whose representatives will visit the hospital and assist us in devising other plans of attack.

  *Relocating the hospital "dumpsters" to an area away from the loading dock. The dumpster is a favorite fly hangout.

  *Imposing a $1 per head charge on all flies who enter the Cafeteria, whether they eat or not.

These measures should help. But before we can claim total victory, we need a total hospital effort. Keep all doors and windows in your area closed, if possible. Avoid direct contact with the enemy, if possible. Report all suggestions concerning this hospital problem to me. And finally, remember that the only good fly is a dead fly!

Thank you for your cooperation and patience.

TS/lm

1063 (7-78)

Exhibit 4.5. Attention-getting memo.

quent miscommunication. When many people must be notified of changes in policies or procedures, of new agency directives or decisions, or of future events, a memo can efficiently do the job. Memos are invaluable when essential information must be passed on to personnel who work flexible hours and alternate shifts, who are employed part-time, or who are on leave or vacation. The memo in Exhibit 4.6 announces an upcoming event to staff members through their department heads. The memo in Exhibit 4.7 informs nursing personnel of an important policy revision.

Certainly, we must remember that memos provide only one-way communication. So when dialogue and feedback are essential to the information being processed, a telephone call or a face-to-face meeting provides a better channel for message communication. But as Norman B. Sigband points out in *Communication for Management and Business,* there are

---

bch
barberton citizens
hospital
Memo

TO: All Department Heads   DATE: November 15, 198_

FROM: Cathy M. Ceccio, R.N., Nursing Education

SUBJECT: Al-Anon "Meeting on Wheels"

Nursing Education is pleased to present an Al-Anon "Meeting on Wheels" on Thursday, November 20, 198_, in the first floor classroom, to all nursing personnel, as well as to all ancillary health care personnel. Because classroom space is limited, please assign some staff members to each time slot.

Scheduled times are as follows:

    November 20, 198_   Thursday   First Floor Classroom

                              1:30 A.M.
                              2:30 A.M.
                          10:00 A.M.
                              1:00 P.M.
                              8:00 P.M.

Al-Anon is a fellowship of men and women who live with or have lived with the problem of alcoholism. The "Meeting on Wheels" will demonstrate the nature of the actual Al-Anon meeting in an abbreviated form, followed by a question-and-answer period. We believe that all health care workers can benefit from this presentation and gain a better understanding of the Al-Anon referral process.

We look forward to seeing you and your staff on November 20. In the meantime, if you have any questions, I'll be glad to answer them. I can be reached at extension 207.

Exhibit 4.6. Informative memo.

four instances when memos can be more appropriate than telephone calls or face-to-face meetings:

1. To transmit *exactly* the same information to several people
2. To put on record the information, policies, or decisions reached at a meeting or conference
3. To confirm, as a matter of record, a decision or agreement
4. To transmit information, policies, or directives to an individual[19]

Staff development instructor Jane Hirsch views the conformation memo (Exhibit 4.8) as an especially valuable tool for nurses in leadership or managerial positions. If it is written soon after the nurse meets with

```
TO:       All Nursing Units              DATE:   January 16, 1981

FROM:     G. Samms, R.N., Infection Control Nurse

SUBJECT:  Surgical Wound Infection Policy



A new policy regarding surgical wound infections has been
reviewed and approved by the Staff Executive Committee.
It reads as follows:

        A patient who develops a post-surgical wound
        infection due to Staphylococcus aureus shall
        not be transferred off the unit to another
        nursing unit.  The proper isolation procedures
        and techniques can be employed on a surgical
        unit as well as on a medical unit.  This will
        eliminate moving the patient, disrupting his
        or her plan of nursing care, and contaminating
        another area of the hospital.

The policy goes into effect on January 30, 1981.  I will be
making rounds on all nursing units during the week of
January 26 to answer your questions.

If you should have any concerns in the meantime, I will be
glad to consult with you.  You can page me or contact me by
phone at extension 671 from 9 a.m. to 5:30 p.m.



G. Samms, R.N., Infection Control Nurse
```

Exhibit 4.7. Informative memo.

```
TO:       Donna McGuire, Blood Bank        DATE:   July 11, 198_
          Supervisor

FROM:     Tish Paulk, R.N., Staff Development, Extension 1160

SUBJECT:  Presentation on Blood Component Therapy to the
          Graduate Nurses


Donna, this note confirms the arrangements we made yesterday
about your presentation on blood component therapy to the new
graduate nurses.  You are scheduled to speak from 1:30-2:30 p.m.
on Wednesday, July 16, in the 4-West Conference Room.  You can
expect approximately 25 persons--15 new nurses plus 10 R.N.s
who have expressed an interest in your talk.  As you requested,
I will bring the overhead projector and the slide projector
to the room at 1:00 p.m., and I will help you set up the room
for your presentation.

Thanks so much for agreeing to speak!  And please call me if
you have any questions or need any other equipment.
```

Exhibit 4.8. Confirmation memo.

another nurse or ancillary department staff member, the memo can confirm specific points of agreement and help prevent misunderstanding and miscommunication. Hirsch suggests that memos conclude with a request for the receiver to contact the sender if his or her understanding varies from that of the sender.[20]

Finally, when you write a memo, try to recall and apply the following key points. First, be direct. Busy readers appreciate getting the main idea first, *then* the necessary details (often itemized in a list), *and then* a courteous, friendly close. But sometimes, especially in bad-news and persuasive situations, you may use the indirect approach in which the big idea is delayed until you first establish a pleasant emotional tone. Second, be complete. Include the specific information (who, what, when, where, why, how) that the receiver needs to know to act on the message. Third, be concise. People respond more favorably to brief, clear memos than to long-winded ones. Fourth, avoid sarcasm. No matter how angry or frustrated you are, keep a negative or irate tone out of your memo. The audience you are addressing may know nothing of the problem that has made you so irritated. Fifth, elicit feedback. Ask your readers to let you know their questions and concerns about your memo. Always indicate how you can be reached.

SUMMARY

Professional nurses in health care agencies will become involved in the formal communication system of the work milieu. Tools that nurses use or develop include committees, agendas, and minutes; procedures and procedure manuals; incident reports; and memos.

A committee is a group of people with a specific purpose who function collectively to attain a goal. Five types of committees in which nurses may participate are standing committees, ad hoc committees or task forces, multidisciplinary committees, advisory committees, and committees based on job function.

Two written tools—the agenda and the minutes—help the committee realize its goals. Agendas are short and written in outline form. They should reflect the chairperson's organizational skills in planning the meeting; thus, items of higher priority should be placed before items of lesser importance. Agendas are usually distributed to committee members several days before the scheduled meeting to remind participants of the meeting and to help them prepare for the meeting.

As the official record of the committee's proceedings, minutes have several purposes. They summarize and record discussion and decisions, note progress toward goals and objectives, and record actions and the delegation of duties. In general, minutes do not have to be excessively detailed.

Procedures are specific, concrete guides to action based on general nursing principles and on agency policies related to the delivery of nursing care. In effect, procedures are the mechanisms or tools to standardize the implementation of agency policies or nursing principles.

Although many recently published procedure references are available for the nurse, most agencies continue to write and compile their own procedure manuals to better reflect their policies and practices. Such manuals are carefully alphabetized, cross-indexed, and placed in a loose-leaf notebook or in a revolving card file.

The exact format for a written procedure does not matter as long as it adequately conveys what the person must do to carry out the procedure effectively, logically, and safely. A procedure format that includes identification, preparation, performance, documentation, and follow-up care helps better incorporate the procedure into client-centered care.

Any successfully written procedure is based on the thorough understanding of a *process,* that is, a specific series of actions that bring about a specific change or result. Process deals with events as they occur in a chronological or sequential fashion. To effectively communicate the procedure's underlying process, the nurse must write understandable instructions. Clear, concise instructions are a prerequisite for being able to perform the process.

Two frequently written messages that nurses write are incident reports and memos. Nurses document incidents, accidents, or unusual occurrences whenever these cause injury or have the potential to harm a client, visitor, or employee. Most incident reports are analytical, for they request observable, factual data, as well as ask the writer to analyze the events that may have led up to, precipitated, or contributed to the incident.

As an integral part of risk management, the incident report is an internal administrative document with the primary purpose of notifying top management of an unusual occurrence. It also serves as a tool for assessing the agency's liability in the event of a lawsuit. The purpose of the incident report is *not* to criticize or discipline but rather to improve care and identify standards for safe client care.

Although an incident may be any unusual occurrence, it usually fits into one of five categories—falls, medication or treatment errors, patient-inherent occurrences, loss of personal effects, and defective equipment or an unsafe environment. The registered nurse and/or the person who discovers the incident will usually complete the documentation.

Agencies use whatever incident report form best meets their needs. The information in the report may be categorized into three separate areas: (1) baseline data, (2) description of the incident and resulting actions taken, and (3) physician's statement. Since the basis of the report is factual information, the nurse avoids ambiguous language and describes the mishap in an orderly, progressive manner, exactly as the events occurred.

Memos are brief internal messages used to transmit information to one person or to an audience of several persons. They may also confirm agreements or decisions reached among participants at meetings. The confirmation memo is a valuable tool of the professional nurse, for it helps prevent miscommunication by documenting in writing specific points of agreement. Because the memo provides only one-way communication, concluding the message by asking for feedback from the audience will help complete the communication loop.

EXERCISES

1. As chairperson of your agency's client education committee, prepare an agenda for next month's meeting. Some of the items the group needs to discuss are the status of the hypertension teaching plan, the evaluation of the pilot project on group diabetic instruction, and the possibility of charging for prenatal nutrition booklets. You also need

to plan time for a report from the chairperson of the community task force.

2. Write the minutes of the client education committee meeting (see the previous exercise). You should add details that are reasonable and likely.

3. From your agency's procedure manual, select a procedure that must be clearly communicated to all levels of nursing personnel and that you believe can be made more effective. Examples of procedures involving all levels of nursing personnel in most agencies include post-mortem care, diabetic urine testing, and application of soft restraints. Rewrite the procedure according to the guidelines given in the text. Evaluate the effectiveness of your writing by asking a newly employed staff member at the agency to demonstrate his or her understanding of the procedure to you.

4. According to the guidelines given in the text, critique and rewrite as necessary the following descriptions of incidents. Use your best judgment in adding appropriate details and deleting ambiguous language.

   a. About 2 o'clock the staff heard a scream—they found Mrs. J. on the floor. She seemed to have tripped over the footstool by her bed. Vital signs within normal range. Doctor called.

   b. Ms. K., a visitor, fell as she got off the elevator. She apparently fell, due to the heel on her sandal coming off. BP 150/90. Stated she was hypertensive. John from Maintenance fixed her shoe. Ms. K. refused to be examined in ER. Walked down hall to see Mrs. C. in room 861. Then, just as visiting hours ended, Ms. K. told aide that her knee really hurt. Aide told unit secretary, who offered to take her to ER. Ms. K. refused again. Stated she was fine.

   c. Mr. T. received an overdose of meperidine—150 mg within 2 hours. I gave him 75 mg IM at 8:45 PM for complaint of generalized abdominal pain. I charted the medication immediately after giving it. But I forgot to sign out for it in the narcotic record. At 10:45 PM Mrs. Western gave Mr. T. an additional dose of 75 mg IM of meperidine since she did not see any medication signed out for him since 4 PM. Physician notified. Vital signs to be monitored every 30 minutes for 6 hours.

   d. Mrs. M. complained of being unable to find eyeglasses. Room searched—glasses not found. Could not remember when she last had them. Nursing supervisor was notified.

5. As secretary of the Gunning College Student Nurses Association, write a memo to all nursing students encouraging them to give blood. The Urbana County Bloodmobile will be on campus in 1 week. Give

specific times and locations. What persuasive talking points will you include to motivate your readers to action?

6. You are head nurse on 2-East, a 30-bed general medical unit. Write a memo to your clinical coordinator confirming the policy you both have agreed on for using volunteers to help transport patients to Radiology and Nuclear Medicine. You decided that a registered nurse will determine which patients may be safely escorted by volunteers. Supply additional details as necessary, including when you agreed on the policy, when it takes effect, and which of you notifies the director of nursing service, the coordinator of volunteers, and the staff of 2-East.

7. Write a memo to the oncology nurse specialist confirming the time, date, place, topic, and audiovisual needs for her inservice presentation to the staffs of three general medical units.

REFERENCES

1. Signe S. Cooper, "Committees That Work," *Journal of Nursing Administration,* 3 (January–February 1973), 31.

2. Cooper, p. 31.

3. Barbara J. Stevens, *First-Line Patient Care Management* (Wakefield, MA: Contemporary Publishing, 1976), p. 170.

4. Lyla Niederbaumer, "Rethinking the Procedure Manual," *Supervisor Nurse,* 8 (April 1977), 59.

5. Barbara J. Stevens, *The Nurse as Executive* (Wakefield, MA: Contemporary Publishing, 1976), p. 110.

6. Genevieve Casanova, "Developing and Writing Policy," *Supervisor Nurse,* 3 (April 1972), 63.

7. Marjorie Moore, "JCAH Standard III: Policies—Guidelines for Action," *Journal of Nursing Administration,* 2 (May–June 1972), 30–31.

8. Niederbaumer, p. 59.

9. Thelma Schwertner and Sue Scibek, "Nursing Care Guidelines," *Supervisor Nurse,* 7 (March 1976), 26.

10. Niederbaumer, p. 59.

11. Margaret L. Wright, "A Lesson in Procedure Writing," *Supervisor Nurse,* 8 (April 1977), 26–27.

12. Sharon Riutta, "Patient-centered Procedures," *Supervisor Nurse,* 7 (April 1976), 30–31.

13. Lillian S. Brunner, "A Guide to Writing Your Policy Manual," *RN,* 37 (April 1974), OR-6.

14. Shannon E. Perry, "Managing to Avoid Malpractice: Part Two," *Journal of Nursing Administration,* 8 (September 1978), 19.

15. Frances H. Lynn, "Incidents—Need They Be Accidents?" *American Journal of Nursing,* 80 (June 1980), 1098.
16. Natalie Slocumb Witte, "Why the Elderly Fall," *American Journal of Nursing,* 79 (November 1979), 1950–1952.
17. Joanna L. Apple, "The Classification of Medication Errors," *Supervisor Nurse,* 7 (December 1976), 23.
18. Lynn, p. 1098.
19. Norman B. Sigband, *Communication for Management and Business,* 2d ed. (Glenview, IL: Scott, Foresman, 1976), p. 372.
20. Jane Hirsch, "When, and How, to Put It in Writing," *RN,* 43 (April 1980), 113.

FURTHER READING

Beaumont, Estelle, and Judy Warmuth. "The New Procedure Reference Manuals." *Nursing79,* 9 (September 1979), 72–77.

Doll, Anne. "What to Do After an Incident." *Nursing80,* 10 (October 1980), 73–79.

Duran, Gladys. "Positive Use of Incident Reports." *Hospitals,* 53 (July 16, 1979), 60, 64, 68.

Ede, Lorice. "The Occupational Safety and Health Act of 1970: Recording and Reporting." *Occupational Health Nursing,* 19 (September 1971), 13–15.

Gryzbek, Tom. "Employee Interest: Key to Successful Incident Reporting System." *Hospitals,* 53 (July 16, 1979), 97–98.

Hershey, Nathan. "Patient Records/Incident Reports." *American Journal of Nursing,* 69 (September 1969), 1931–1932.

Josehart, Harold E. "Developing a Hospital Policy and Procedure Manual." *AORN Journal,* 19 (February 1974), 498–516.

Matthies, Leslie H. *The Playscript Procedure: A New Tool of Administration.* Stamford, CT: Office Publications, 1961.

Salman, Steven L. "Committee Is an Important Tool in Risk Management." *Hospitals,* 54 (Sept. 16, 1980), 45, 48, 50.

Stevens, Beulah. "The Playscript Method of Developing Administrative Procedures." *Supervisor Nurse,* 6 (June 1975), 40–42, 44–45.

Webster, Eric. "Memo Mania: Its Causes, Carriers, and Cures." *Management Review,* 56 (September 1967), 32–36.

Wrenn, Alta J. "The Incident Report as a Risk Mangement Tool." *Supervisor Nurse,* 12 (January 1981), 34–35.

CHAPTER V

Writing and
the Nurse Leader

Objectives

After studying this chapter, you will be able to

1. State the characteristics of justification reports that use the direct approach or the indirect approach.
2. Write justification reports using both the direct approach and the indirect approach.
3. State the four components of a brief informal proposal.
4. Discuss the six components of longer, unsolicited proposals.
5. Draft a proposal to improve or change a specific element in your agency's health care delivery system.
6. Explain the components of the written job description.
7. Evaluate the effectiveness of selected job descriptions.
8. Discuss the relationship between the written job description and the performance appraisal tool.
9. State the three key elements of the performance appraisal process.
10. Discuss the purposes of the performance appraisal.
11. Discuss the difference between performance appraisals based on personality traits and those based on performance standards.
12. Write clear performance standards.
13. Write meaningful anecdotal notes based on observable behavior or performance.
14. Write letters of appreciation, praise, and good will.

As professional nurses take on leadership roles, they become more and more concerned with the problem-solving process and with effecting change through persuasion. As you will recall from our discussion early in the first chapter, the higher up you go in an organization, the more time you will likely spend communicating—and that means a good deal of writing. At this point, therefore, we are ready to delve more deeply into the formal communication system of the work milieu. This chapter helps nurse leaders successfully plan and write justification reports, proposals, job descriptions, performance appraisals, and letters of appreciation, praise, and good will.

JUSTIFICATION REPORTS

Nurses in leadership positions must frequently write requests justifying new equipment or supplies, increased staffing, or additional space. With the cost of supplies, equipment, and labor escalating yearly in the health care field, budgets in many agencies cannot possibly support all the demands that are made on them. In many agencies, therefore, obtaining new and replacement equipment, adding to staff, remodeling the work or client care environment, and securing more space must be formally requested and justified. Your written request may appear in memo format, although sometimes letter format is used.

After nursing administration and the chief fiscal officer study written requests, nurses may be asked to defend their requests in person before financial committee members. But it is often the written justification itself that persuades the administrator to allocate funds for the nursing department's new equipment or project instead of for some other purpose. Effective communication *can* make a difference.

Two Approaches to Justification Reports

There are two ways to organize and present justification reports—directly and indirectly. The *direct approach* is appropriate when the writer anticipates few problems or little resistance in securing the request. Direct requests are immediate messages with the following characteristics:

1. They immediately make the request.
2. They then develop the rationale or persuasive explanation for the request.
3. They conclude by summarizing supporting arguments, reiterating reader and/or agency benefits, and encouraging a prompt response or setting a suitable target date.

The nurse writing a justification report with the direct approach expects that the reader of the message is already motivated to grant the request. For example, if a hospital's philosophy embraces the concept of family-centered maternity care, it is likely that funds will be allocated for a birthing room. Perhaps the nurse leader and representatives from nursing administration have talked informally about remodeling one of the traditional delivery rooms into a homelike birthing room. The consensus is favorable. An ad hoc committee may be formed to pursue the project. After investigating and deliberating, the committee may write a formal justification report in memo format and with the direct approach. Indeed, agreement to fund the remodeling may have been tacitly given by administration during the planning stage; so the formal justification report may be considered "for the record" by the administrator. As a result, the direct, or straightforward, approach can be successfully employed in this communication situation.

The justification report in Exhibit 5.1 uses the direct approach in making a reasoned request for a classroom in an unoccupied old wing of a medium-size city hospital. Because the old wing is no longer suitable for client care, most rooms there now store miscellaneous equipment. The project co-directors of the Adult Nurse Practitioner program send their special request to the assistant administrator responsible for allocating space. Since space is not a problem at their agency, the nurses decide to write directly. Both the subject line and the first paragraph of the memo

```
DATE:     November 30, 1980

TO:       Kenneth Roser, Assistant Administrator

FROM:     DeAnne Schlutt and Sarah Altieri
          Project Co-Directors, Adult Nurse Practitioner Program

SUBJECT:  Classroom Request for the Adult Nurse Practitioner Program


We request that Metropolitan Hospital's Adult Nurse Practitioner (ANP)
program have its own classroom in the north wing of the old hospital.
Room 631 would be especially suitable since it is large and is away
from other offices on the wing.  Its location would help insure the
privacy that students need while learning and practicing physical
assessment skills.

The reasons we need a separate classroom for nurse practitioner
students are integrally related to the scope of Metropolitan Hospital's
ANP program.  During the first 12 weeks of the 26-week program, nurse
practitioner students will participate in formal classes or independent
study eight hours a day.  The first 12 weeks are crucial--the students
will be learning basic physical assessment, a rigorous discipline
that demands a quiet, private environment.  Students will use the
classroom as a learning laboratory, practicing their newly acquired
skills on each other before using them on patient care units.

The students in the ANP program will be using a wide variety of
audiovisual equipment--videotape monitors, slide-tape projectors,
16 mm. projectors, dictaphones, and tape recorders.  Having a separate
classroom will enable the students to use audiovisual equipment and
manikin training simulators in independent study at any time of the
day.  It will also provide a place for the students to store the other
equipment they use to learn physical assessment skills--books, journals,
stethoscopes, ophthalmoscopes, otoscopes,  tuning forks, preference
notebooks, and clinical observation notebooks.

After students complete the first 12 weeks of the ANP program, they
will continue to need their own classroom.  Nurses will accompany
their nurse and physician preceptors on morning rounds, and a quiet
classroom will provide the right environment to help them prepare
for their clinical practice experience.  Advanced classes in
pathophysiology, EKG interpretation, and cardiac life support will
be held in the afternoon.
```

Exhibit 5.1. Justification report using the direct approach.

In short, room 631 on the north wing of the old hospital would be
ideal for Metro's ANP program. Its location will help insure the
quiet and privacy so necessary for learning and practicing physical
assessment skills and other advanced clinical nursing courses. And
the room is large enough to provide adequate storage for all the
equipment and learning resource materials which the program demands.

Since we anticipate the starting date of the ANP program as
February 1, 1981, may we have your response by December 15? If
you have any questions regarding the program or our request, we
would be most willing to discuss them with you. We can be reached
at extension 128.

Exhibit 5.1. (Continued)

make explicit this message's main point. The second, third, and fourth
paragraphs develop the case with specific details and agency-related benefits. The next-to-last paragraph summarizes the arguments supporting
the request. The writers conclude by encouraging a prompt response and
by telling the reader how they can be reached.

Although the direct approach is appropriate for justification reports
when the nurse does not expect resistance from the reader, the *indirect
approach* tends to be more effective when the writer needs to gain support
from someone who may resist or who may have little initial interest in
the request.

The indirect, or delayed, strategy calls for an opening or buffer paragraph that gets in step with the reader by tying in the eventual request
with the receiver's other interests or projects. In the indirect approach,
then, the writer delays the actual request until late in the message. The
four-part plan is (1) to arouse the reader's interest or acknowledge his or
her cooperation in a related project, (2) to develop a careful rationale in
support of the unstated but implicit request, (3) to make the request and
elaborate with as many details as necessary for the particular reader, and
(4) to provide a positive, courteous closing statement.

Let us suppose that the project co-directors of the Adult Nurse Practitioner program just discussed faced a different communication situation.
Instead of space being relatively plentiful at their institution, let us assume that the circumstances have changed. Now very few rooms are
available in the old north wing because the scope of the agency's ancillary
services has grown and many new departments have moved into former
client rooms, converting them into comfortable offices. In addition, the
assistant administrator responsible for allocating and monitoring space
has not granted nursing service's requests for additional space in the recent past. With these variables in mind, the co-directors need to draft an

appropriately persuasive message. This time, however, choosing the indirect approach and perhaps using letter format (to avoid a memo's rather too obvious subject line) would seem the better strategy.

The indirectly planned justification letter in Exhibit 5.2 arouses the reader's interest at the outset. It also acknowledges his support of a related project, namely, the Family Practice Residency program. This is you-attitude in action. The four paragraphs after the first develop the ration-

---

November 30, 1980

Dear Mr. Roser:

We were pleased to attend your presentation on the
nurse-physician-administrator relationship at the last
Executive Committee Meeting. After hearing you discuss how you
expect the Adult Nurse Practitioner students will interrelate with
physicians in Metropolitan Hospital's Family Practice Residency
program, we know you are eager to see us establish our first
Adult Nurse Practitioner (ANP) program. We heartily concur with
the main point of your presentation--not only will the ANP
program attract more and better qualified nurses, but it will also
provide one more "selling point" to attract highly qualified
physicians to the Family Practice Residency program.

Like the Family Practice Residency program, the ANP program will
have a rigorous curriculum. And we want the program to be one that
all of us at Metropolitan Hospital can be proud of.

During the first 12 weeks of the 26-week program, ANP students will
participate in formal classes or independent study eight hours a
day. The first 12 weeks of the program are essential to the
practitioners' future success, for during this time they will be
learning basic physical assessment skills. This is a rigorous
discipline demanding a quiet, private environment.

The ANP students will use a learning laboratory to practice their
beginning skills on each other before using them on patient care
units. They will also use a variety of audiovisual equipment (such
as videotape machines, slide-tape projectors, 16 mm. projectors,
and tape recorders) and manikin training simulators to help them
master assessment skills. In addition, they will accumulate a variety
of books, journals, charts, clinical observation notebooks, as well
as ophthalmoscopes, otoscopes, sensitive dual-head stethoscopes,
and tuning forks.

After the beginning physical assessment modules are completed, ANP
students will begin to accompany physician preceptors on patient
rounds. Some of the preceptors will be physicians enrolled in the
Family Practice Residency program. We expect that nurse practitioner
students will need to devote considerable time to preparation for
making rounds with the preceptors. After rounds are completed, we
anticipate that students will need to study independently in preparation

---

Exhibit 5.2. Justification report using the indirect approach.

for future clinical experiences as well as for classes in advanced
cardiac life support, pathophysiology, and EKG interpretation.

Room 631 on the north wing of the old hospital should provide a
quiet, private environment for the ANP program. The room is large
enough to accommodate desks, examination tables, audiovisual
equipment, and other learning resources which the program demands.

Since we plan to begin the first ANP program on February 1, 1981,
may we have your response to our request for room 631 by December 15?
If you have any questions regarding our request, please contact us
at extension 128.

Sincerely,

Exhibit 5.2. (Continued)

ale for getting a classroom, but the writers do not specifically make the
request until the sixth paragraph. By that point, as you can see, the
groundwork has been laid and the request comes as a logical conclusion
to all that has preceded it. The closing paragraph shows courtesy, sets a
response date and justifies it, and offers to answer any questions.

Another Example

The directly planned justification memo in Exhibit 5.3, written by a head
nurse to a nursing administrator, suggests a way to save money by purchasing the more convenient and efficiently organized prepackaged
dressing kits available from Pharmex. In such reports, writers try to
solve problems they observe on the clinical unit. Notice the effective use
of headings and the centered table, two features that greatly enhance this
short report's readability.

Exhibit 5.3. A directly planned justification memo.

DATE: February 4, 1981
TO: Mariane Kopek, R.N., M.S.N., Director of Surgical Nursing
FROM: Gail W. Easterling, R.N., Head Nurse, 7-North
SUBJECT: How Prepackaged Hyperalimentation Dressing Change Kits Would Save at Least
          $800 a Year

Purpose

To save Green County Hospital at least $800 a year, I suggest that we start stocking
prepackaged hyperalimentation dressing change kits in Central Service.

Cost and Savings

Sterile dressing change kits, prepackaged exactly to GCH's specifications, are available from
Pharmex Medical Supply Company. The cost is $3.20 per kit, which can be reduced 20% (or
$.65 per kit, to $2.55) when at least 500 kits are purchased at a time. Since the average

Exhibit 5.3. (Continued)

daily census of clients requiring hyperalimentation dressing changes is 9, GCH would use approximately 270 kits per month. So it would be realistic to order 500 kits at a time to be eligible for the 20% discount.

The current cost of individually purchased supplies used in daily hyperalimentation dressing changes is as follows:

Item	Cost
1 pr. sterile scissors (from disposable suture set)	$1.07
1 prepackaged sterile T dressing	.45
2 pr. sterile gloves @ $.17	.34
2 prepackaged sterile 4 × 4's @ $.08	.16
1 package povidone iodine ointment	.15
2 prepackaged sterile acetone swabs @ $.09	.18
1 prepackaged sterile tincture of benzoin swab	.10
1 elastic dressing, 4" × 3"	.35
	$2.80

By purchasing 500 Pharmex hyperalimentation dressing change kits at a time, we can realize a savings of $.25 per kit. That amounts to $67.50 a month, or $810 a year.

Procedure

We will follow the same procedure as we do currently in evaluating any new product or equipment. Jerry Jackson, purchasing agent, will ask the Pharmex sales representative to demonstrate his firm's prepackaged hyperalimentation dressing kit to the product utilization committee at the March 14 meeting. If two-thirds of the committee agree that the quality of the product is as good as 80% of the individually prepackaged items that the hospital now stocks for use in hyperalimentation dressing changes, Mr. Jackson will negotiate a 120-day trial contract with Pharmex. The contract would take effect April 15 and be up for renewal after August 12.

Between July 5 and July 15, nurses who have used the Pharmex hyperalimentation dressing kits will complete a "New Product Evaluation Survey" (Form No. 137B) and send their appraisal to Mr. Jackson. The results will be tallied, summarized, and presented to the product utilization committee at the July 29 meeting. Based on the evaluation survey, committee members will determine if the quality of the Pharmex product justifies the savings.

Recommendation and Additional Information

I recommend that we start using the Pharmex hyperalimentation dressing change kit because of its significant direct savings to Green County Hospital.

Furthermore, based on a small preliminary study of six nurses who did hyperalimentation dressing changes, the three who used the Pharmex kit saved approximately 3 minutes in gathering the equipment as compared to those who used separately packaged equipment to perform the dressing change. And because the kits are efficiently packaged, the three nurses who used the Pharmex kit saved an additional 1.5 minutes in performing the actual dressing change as compared to the other three nurses who did the dressing change using the supplies we presently stock.

The potential savings in nursing time during the procedure could amount to an additional *$.20* per dressing change when the average staff nurse's hourly salary ($8.25) is divided by the decrease in nursing time (1.5 minutes). Although this time-study sample was small, this could amount to a monthly savings of $54 in nursing salaries—or *$648* a year.

PROPOSALS

The difference between justification reports and proposals may seem small, yet the distinction is worth making. Justification reports tend to present a single, somewhat limited problem (as opposed to a more general or global one in proposals), together with data to justify a recommended solution. Proposals, on the other hand, are persuasive reports that attempt to gain authorization for a specific and significant course of action. Internally generated proposals developed by one person or by several people working together, for example, deal with changes that could significantly alter one or more parts of the organization. Proposals may deal with such big issues as establishing a new program, altering the delivery of client care, or undertaking a research project—just about any significant process that the proposal writer believes would benefit the agency. In short, when contrasted with justification reports, proposals are the means for suggesting far-reaching, more global ideas for improving the health care delivery system.

Proposals may be classified according to audience, length and complexity, degree of formality, and whether they are solicited or unsolicited. Internal proposals are generated within the agency; external proposals are generated from outside the agency. Proposals may be short (three pages or fewer) or long (four pages or more), simple in scope or quite complex. Solicited proposals are "asked for," that is, written in response to a formal or informal request for a proposal. Unsolicited proposals are initiated by the proposal writer.

Although internal proposals are generally unsolicited, external proposals may often be solicited by management or administration. Thus, a health care facility may formally issue a request for a proposal to outside consulting firms to conduct research on the system of health care delivery used at the facility. Several consulting firms in nursing systems analysis might respond, then, each with a specific proposal on how it would conduct the study that the facility wants done.

When nurses in leadership positions become involved in writing proposals, they usually write internal unsolicited proposals. Whether these are short or long, simple or complex depends on factors such as the nature and scope of the proposal. For proposals dealing with large projects or complex research studies, many people may collaborate on the plan. Later, one person may do the actual writing, compiling the input from other members of the proposal committee.

Proposal writers should constantly keep in mind whether a proposal was solicited or not. Consulting firms that write proposals in response to a health care facility's request for a proposal do not have to prove that there is a need for the services they can provide. Since the health care agency has already acknowledged this need, the writers of solicited proposals have only to focus on persuading the agency that their firm is the best one for solving the agency's problem. In unsolicited proposals, however, it is essential for nurse writers to convince the audience that a need exists for the project they are proposing. If writers of unsolicited proposals cannot convince their audience of this need from the very beginning, the audience will see no particular value in the services or project being proposed. And the remainder of the proposal will go unread.

Memo format is appropriate for informal internal proposals of three pages or fewer. Brief informal proposals should include (1) the concept being advanced, (2) the rationale, (3) the method of implementation, and (4) the conclusions and benefits. But when the length of the proposal reaches four pages or more, a modified report format should be used to help proposal writers more clearly develop their ideas. Moreover, appropriate heading categories enable busy proposal readers to follow the report more easily.

We recommend the following six components for unsolicited internal proposals of four pages or more. Naturally, the proposal writer might need to adapt this format, too, depending on the nature of the proposal.

1. Introduction
   1.1 Purpose
   1.2 Statement of the problem or need
   1.3 Background of the problem or need
   1.4 Scope of the proposal
2. Process or methodology
3. Management of tasks or objectives
   3.1 Task analysis
   3.2 Time frame for implementation
   3.3 Availability of personnel, facilities, space, equipment
4. Financial considerations
   4.1 Capital budget expenditures (remodeling, new equipment, additional staff, etc.)
   4.2 Operating budget expenditures
   4.3 Potential savings
5. Personnel qualifications
6. Conclusions

As the preceding outline reveals, the introduction immediately provides the pertinent information that the reader needs to know about the problem in order to appreciate the proposal's importance. After supplying the proposal's purpose, the introduction treats the problem or need with which the proposal is concerned and any pertinent background. The scope statement defines the proposal's boundaries. Thus, if the proposal discusses establishing primary nursing at an acute care agency, the scope statement tells whether the proposal will be limited to a pilot project on one nursing unit, to one division of related nursing units (such as all general medical units), or to all nursing units in the agency. At times, too, it may be helpful to state precisely what is *not* included.

The body of the proposal, represented by the second through the fifth items in our outline, elaborates on how to implement the proposal, the time frame for accomplishing specific tasks, and the order in which they are to be done. It pays to be realistic about the time frame, for one common mistake that proposal writers make is underestimating how long it will take to implement a project. Reviewing the availability of personnel, facilities, space, and equipment is also essential. Costs, both direct and indirect, and potential savings should be addressed honestly. Finally, the body of the proposal should contain the qualifications of those personnel who will be involved in the project, directly connecting their educational and experiential backgrounds to their ability to succeed in the new endeavor.

The concluding section reviews the main points and reasons for accepting the proposal. If the writer has written effectively, clearly defining the problem and supporting the proposal with well-substantiated arguments, this last part is easy to write. Here the writer may employ several last-minute strategies to persuade the reader to accept the proposal—perhaps stating a willingness to be available for a follow-up interview or even to modify the proposal.

Other items that may be included in a proposal, especially if it is long, are a title page, a table of contents, an abstract, and relevant attachments such as diagrams describing physical or managerial changes. The title page contains the exact title of the proposal, the author's name, the date, and the receiver's name. The table of contents, listing the proposal's topics and any illustrations, gives the page numbers on which they can be found. The abstract, a 100 to 200-word synopsis of the proposal, precedes the introduction. Valuable in summarizing the contents of long proposals, abstracts make it possible for readers to gain an overview of the proposal.

We think this necessarily brief discussion of proposals can help you when you are called on to draft a proposal.

JOB DESCRIPTIONS

If there is one task that nurses in leadership or managerial positions dislike doing almost as much as writing and giving employee performance appraisals, it is writing and revising job descriptions. Yet accurate, up-to-date job descriptions provide a means for implementing the health care organization's philosophy, purpose, and objectives. Although final responsibility for seeing that adequate job descriptions are maintained lies with the nurse executive in nursing administration, nurses in various leadership positions play key roles in helping to determine how well the written job descriptions reflect what nursing personnel at different levels actually do in their daily activities.

Background and Advantages

Nurse leaders may become aware of how effective their agency's job descriptions are when they are asked to help write a job description for a newly created position. As they review the descriptions of already established positions, they can consider how accurately each description fits the organizational reality. A head nurse who wishes to justify a merit raise for a staff nurse may turn to the job description to verify that the nurse is performing above the standards set forth in the document. Staff development instructors use job descriptions to orient new employees to the agency's expectations about their job duties and responsibilities. And those involved in interviewing applicants for positions use the job description to determine how well a potential employee fits the opening. Likewise, the candidate who has an opportunity to read the job description can see precisely what the position entails.

Job descriptions seem to become outdated quickly at many facilities, but this is probably because they are not systematically reviewed every year. The chief characteristic of outdated job descriptions is the disparity between the idealized write-up and the "real world" job activities. "Perhaps nurses and other nursing personnel would reap more job satisfaction if job descriptions truly reflected job functions and responsibilities,"[1] note the authors of a recent *Supervisor Nurse* article. Of course, although job descriptions should reflect what nurses in various positions actually do and are responsible for, they should also be flexible enough to encourage creativity.

One definition of the term *job description* that we find helpful is "a written word picture of organizational relationships, responsibilities, and specific duties that constitute a given job."[2] In addition, the job description should objectively relate the vital elements of the position, including scope, authority, and place in the organizational hierarchy. Components of the job description are

- Department
- Job title
- Date

- Job summary
- Responsibilities
- Job specifications

The advantages of maintaining updated job descriptions are many:

1. They help reduce role ambiguity and foster role clarity among nursing personnel in regard to the delivery of client care.
2. They refine and clarify the organizational structure, specifically delineating the chain of command.
3. They provide objective information on which to base salary scales. Thus, the position with increased authority and responsibility can be placed higher in the salary scale distribution without managers having to rely on judging personality traits.
4. They describe jobs but avoid describing people's personalities.
5. They can furnish an objective basis for evaluating employee performance.
6. They state the areas of freedom, flexibility, and creativity that are permitted for certain positions.

Writing the Job Description

The purpose of writing a job description is to put clearly in writing an explicit statement of the duties and responsibilities for anyone who is hired for the position. While the job description is a summary in brief of the job, it is not associated with the personal characteristics of any particular employee.

In writing a job description, you should focus on the job summary, responsibilities, and job specifications sections. Just how well have you written these critical components? Are they comprehensible to people both within and outside of the nursing department? Are they specific enough so that people understand what they are to do, yet flexible enough to cover logically related (but unforeseen) job responsibilities? Have you analyzed the duties and responsibilities carefully to be sure that those items actually assigned to the job description do, indeed, belong there?

The job summary section of the Nurse Clinician job description (Exhibit 5.4) reviews the position's scope and elements. This section usually appears in paragraph form and complete sentences. It often reflects nursing service philosophy, and sometimes it restates the philosophy in abbreviated form.

Exhibit 5.4. Job description for Nurse Clinician.

Department: Nursing Service
Job Title: Nurse Clinician
Date: June 1, 1981

Job Summary

The Nurse Clinician is directly responsible to the Director of Nursing Service or her designee and works under the medical supervision of physicians who have signed a written agreement to participate in the Clinician Program. The Nurse Clinician promotes a coordinated, interdisciplinary working relationship with physicians, nursing staff, and other members of the health care team. She/he provides clinical nursing leadership, serving as a role model for the professional registered nurse by assessing, planning, coordinating, and evaluating client care activities. The Clinician performs clinically advanced procedures and documents them as directed by the physician. She/he accepts responsibility for instituting appropriate measures to meet client needs according to physician preferences.

Responsibilities

1. The Nurse Clinician is responsible for promoting a coordinated, interdisciplinary relationship with physicians, nursing staff, and other members of the health care team.
    1.1 Makes rounds with assigned physicians no less than twice a week in order to develop a thorough understanding of the client's history, present illness, and related progress.
    1.2 Relates knowledge of the client's clinical data and progress to appropriate nursing personnel.
2. The Nurse Clinician provides clinical nursing leadership and serves as a role model for the professional registered nurse.
    2.1 Assists nursing personnel in the evaluation of clinical data and findings, suggesting appropriate follow-up care.
    2.2 Assesses the client's condition regarding nursing care and medical progress, including psychosocial needs.
3. The Nurse Clinician coordinates and evaluates client care activities.
    3.1 Recognizes priority needs of clients and reports significant clinical data to the physician by reviewing the clinical data results, evaluating the clinical picture the client presents, and ordering additional clinical data to follow up the present problem, according to standing orders.
    3.2 Performs health histories and physical assessments on all clients admitted under the medical management of physicians who are participating in the program.
    3.3 Recognizes potentially serious conditions and takes appropriate action to avert irreversible conditions, according to standing orders.
4. The Nurse Clinician promotes and assists with client/family teaching and assists the physician with discharge instructions.
    4.1 Promotes the use of educational resources such as preop teaching classes, standardized teaching care plans, selected audiovisual materials, and the Health Education Television Network.
    4.2 Provides reinforcement of home care instructions.
    4.3 Provides medical discharge instructions as delegated by the physician.
5. The Nurse Clinician maintains intradepartmental communications by attending selected meetings, such as Head Nurse and/or Supervisor meetings.
6. The Nurse Clinician participates in the instruction of basic cardiac life support, as needed. She/he responds to and participates in all emergency codes while on duty.

Exhibit 5.4. (Continued)

7. The Nurse Clinician performs clinically advanced procedures and documents them appropriately.

   7.1 Administers specifically ordered intravenous medications, according to the agency's policies, procedures, and standing orders.

   7.2 Documents and signs appropriate progress notes such as changes in the client's general condition, special procedures performed, and the results of pertinent data as reflected by the client's condition.

   7.3 Performs clinically advanced procedures as directed by the physician and as delineated on the Nurse Clinician Procedure List.

   7.4 Assists the physician and staff nurses with the insertion of subclavian lines and chest tubes.

   7.5 Initiates orders for diagnostic tests, including (but not limited to) complete blood counts, routine urinalyses, electrocardiograms, blood sugars, electrolytes, and arterial blood gasses.

8. The Nurse Clinician performs as a clinical nursing consultant to all areas of Nursing Service.

   8.1 Provides clinical nursing consultant services, only as requested by unit staff nurses, on all in-house clients whose physicians are not participating in the Nurse Clinician Program.

   8.2 Provides clinical nursing consultant leadership in the administration of client care by assisting in the recognition of educational needs of the nursing staff for procedures and/or clinical nursing problems.

   8.3 Assists in the development of closer communication between client, physician, and staff.

9. The Nurse Clinician accepts responsibility for instituting appropriate measures to meet client needs according to physician preferences. She/he writes additional orders and performs special functions as directed by physicians according to established agency policy and as permitted by Illinois licensure in the practice of professional nursing.

Job Specifications

1. *Experience*

   Current clinical experience in an acute care agency with at least 1 year current work experience. Demonstrates the potential for superior competence in clinical nursing skills and judgments. Demonstrates ability to adapt to changing clinical situations with a logical and reasonable approach. Possesses finesse in dealing with other members of the health care team. Displays initiative in recognizing problems and willingness to assume responsibility for appropriate follow-up care.

2. *Education*

   Graduate of a state-approved school of professional nursing with current license to practice nursing in Illinois. Must satisfactorily complete 6 months in the Clinician Orientation Program, after which the Clinician must be capable of performing required job responsibilities independently. Each Clinician is responsible for participating in and/or attending 20 contact hours of continuing education per year. Individual participation is encouraged through seminars and workshops. Previous experience in critical care and/or nursing management is helpful.

3. *Dexterity*

   Must understand and be capable of working with sophisticated equipment and diagnostic tools. Must possess sound communication skills to coordinate client care by physicians, nursing staff, ancillary departments, and families. Must possess teaching skills to guide staff, teach clients, and plan for discharge instructions.

Exhibit 5.4. (Continued)

4. *Character of Supervision Received*

   Performs under the direct medical supervision of participating physicians in the Clinician Program. Client care provided is usually performed independently with follow-up of progress by peers, nursing staff, and attending physicians. Problems are referred directly to the Director of Nursing Service and/or the Physician Advisor.

5. *Character of Supervision Given*

   Assumes direct responsibility for clinical nursing care provided on all participating physicians' services. Provides consultant-type clinical supervision for all in-house clients. Initiates various client treatments, tests, and procedures as directed by participating physicians. Acts as a clinical coordinator of client care between medical staff, client, and nursing staff.

6. *Responsibility for Interpersonal Relationships*

   Must be able to establish and maintain excellent rapport with physicians, clients, and agency staff, or results of duties performed may be seriously damaged or useless. Sets a clinical example for all nursing staff. Must perform functions with a high degree of character and integrity. Must be willing to work with everyone in a cooperative manner and be willing to explain logic behind actions when asked.

7. *Pressure of Work*

   Extremely high pressure when making clinical judgments and/or meeting needs. Must be capable of and responsible for making appropriate decisions, taking action, and providing follow-up care and yet function within the guidelines of her/his license to practice nursing. Must understand own limitations professionally, legally, and morally, and be prepared to refuse to perform any duty or function that is not within her/his scope or ability.

8. *Unusual Working Conditions*

   Excellent physical stamina is required to provide services to clients located on various units throughout the agency. Frequently called in emergency situations. Must learn to establish appropriate priorities.

As you can see from the Nurse Clinician job description, the long responsibilities section appears in outline form. Each main responsibility is stated in a complete sentence; however, each discrete task begins with a specific verb that focuses on the employee's performance.

The job specifications section is divided into appropriate heading categories such as experience, education, dexterity, and unusual working conditions. Intentional sentence fragments may suffice here, for the specifications apply to the job or to the person who holds the job.

PERFORMANCE APPRAISALS

Nurses in leadership positions frequently find themselves participating in performance reviews, that is, giving formal oral and written evaluations to employees to inform them of how well they are doing their jobs. To be sure, well-written, explicitly phrased job descriptions aid the performance appraisal process. If the job descriptions are free from ambiguity, it is much easier for the employer to determine how well employees are doing their jobs.

Purposes and Standards

There is often a good deal of documentation that the nurse leader must do during the performance appraisal. The actual writing will vary, however, according to the institution's performance appraisal tool, its performance review policies and procedures, and the degree to which the employee meets the job standards. And although documentation clearly stating to what extent the employee meets the job standards is essential to the success of the evaluation process, the *total* performance appraisal process actually requires three key elements: (1) the written evaluation based on objective work standards, (2) the feedback interview or meeting, and (3) the goal-planning session between the superior and the employee.[3]

Formal, systematic performance appraisals serve many purposes. Probably the most important purpose is to let employees know where they stand, for regularly scheduled performance reviews give them the opportunity to hear from their immediate supervisors just how well they are doing. Related to this primary purpose of knowing where one stands is the basic premise on which performance appraisals are based. Thus, in Susan Albrecht's words, "the act of being appraised of positive qualities and shortcomings, and consequently knowing where one stands with one's 'boss,' will stimulate improvement of an employee's performance."[4] And so the review process can be a powerful incentive and reinforcer—in short, a significant tool at the nurse leader's disposal to improve the quality of care that employees give to their clients. Other purposes of performance reviews range from discovering who deserves a promotion to detecting who is doing poor work to fostering better supervisor-subordinate communication.

Although the review process consists of three interdependent elements, much discussion centers on the evaluation form that the agency uses. Bureaucratic pressures often encourage nurse leaders to view the performance appraisal as nothing more than a "paper" requirement, another form to complete within a specified period. But nothing could be further from the truth. Most personnel experts agree that it is not the specific rating form that guarantees the success of the performance appraisal; rather, it is the face-to-face communication that occurs in the feedback interview and in the goal-setting session between supervisor and employee that makes the whole process so beneficial.

So much discussion may center on the performance appraisal tool, however, perhaps because it is a difficult task to accurately evaluate another's job performance. Traditional evaluation forms have focused on employees' personality traits rather than on objective, observable performance, thus making it even more difficult for supervisors and nurse leaders to give meaningful evaluations. A traditional form might include such descriptive categories of personality traits as attendance, punctuality, appearance, attitude toward job, cooperation, dependability, judgment, initiative, and resourcefulness.

If a numerical-descriptive rating scale is associated with each trait or quality, it may become very difficult to evaluate the employee. For example, if a new graduate nurse is being evaluated on her resourcefulness by her clinical nurse preceptor, the juxtaposition of a numerical rating scale and the specific trait may cause confusion. If a rating of "1" is considered significantly below average and a rating of "5" is considered significantly above average, the preceptor may rate the average new graduate nurse as an average "3" in resourcefulness. But such a rating on such a scale gives no real indication of just what "average" resourcefulness is.

On the other hand, when the performance appraisal tool identifies the categories to be rated in terms of performance standards, the written portion of the evaluation becomes much more meaningful. Instead of being rated on personality traits, the nurse is now evaluated according to whether she or he meets the standards of performance for the job. Performance standards are identifiable, measurable achievement criteria that signify a level or baseline against which to measure an action or event. A primary nurse might be evaluated on the following performance components that appear in the agency's job description for a primary nurse:

- Assessing
- Planning
- Implementing
- Evaluating
- Teaching clients and family
- Directing and coordinating others
- Making decisions

Clearly, these elements differ greatly from those categories of personality traits such as attendance, appearance, and initiative.

How are specific performance standards developed and written? Consider the following six standards for a primary nurse that appear under the major job function of "Directing and Coordinating Others":

1. Communicates to co-workers, orally and in writing, the plan of care and nursing orders
2. Interprets the nursing assessment and plan of care to other members of the nursing staff and interdisciplinary health team
3. Directs the activities and personnel on the unit in the head nurse's absence
4. Evaluates the performance of co-workers in relation to job expectations and responsibilities
5. Coordinates services that affect client care, such as radiology, occupational therapy, and physical therapy
6. Seeks help from appropriate resource persons when unusual or difficult management problems occur

Notice that these performance standards, like behavioral or performance

Exhibit 5.5. Head Nurse Performance Standards: Communication.

Explanation of Rating Scale: 1—Meets standard: consistently performs at the level the standard describes.
2—Exceeds standard: performs at a higher level than the standard describes.
3—Does not meet standard: does not meet the level of performance the standard describes.
4—Standard not now applicable.

	Rating	Comments
1. Maintains a professional relationship with staff, other departments, and physicians	_____	_____
2. Acts on interdepartmental problems, attempting to resolve them	_____	_____
3. Implements physicians' orders appropriately	_____	_____
4. Reports promptly changes in client status to appropriate staff members	_____	_____
5. Provides a mechanism for giving staff a written and oral report on their assigned clients	_____	_____
6. Conducts monthly unit meetings for all staff to share information and to facilitate problem solving	_____	_____
7. Communicates accurately and promptly changes in agency policies and corrects misinterpretations	_____	_____
8. Writes clearly understood reports, memos, and minutes	_____	_____
9. Conducts scheduled meetings with staff to inform them of administrative decisions that concern them	_____	_____
10. Schedules meetings with the nurse manager once a month to discuss progress toward the accomplishment of unit and managerial goals	_____	_____

---

objectives, focus on the nurse's performance—not on nebulously defined personality traits. The verbs that begin each standard are active and specific. Even though each standard cannot be quantitatively measured, each standard attempts to describe the minimal level of competence that personnel must demonstrate to prove they are accomplishing this aspect of the job.

Performance appraisal tools that combine a standard-oriented rating scale with carefully conceived performance standards can be very effective. But there should also be adequate space for the evaluator's comments to clarify or elaborate on those standards that the employee exceeds or does not meet. Exhibit 5.5 shows communication performance standards for a head nurse position together with an appropriately useful rating scale.

Anecdotal Notes

In concluding this part of the discussion, we need to mention that anecdotal notes can be a valuable device at the nurse leader's disposal for recording a variety of objective descriptions about an employee's performance. They can be used to document behavior that exceeds the accepted work standard, does not meet the standard, or requires disciplinary action. Usually, anecdotal notes are recorded in narrative form on plain paper. But they may also be written on a loosely structured form, using either a narrative or a combination of a narrative and concise phrases.

The anecdotal note, advises Ann Marriner, should clearly state who performed the specific behavior, who observed that behavior or event, and the time, date, and place that it occurred. The incident itself and related environmental factors make up the bulk of the documentation. Although the nurse may make specific interpretations and recommendations about the observed behavior, Marriner suggests that "value laden words such as good and bad . . . be avoided."[5]

The main advantage of anecdotal notes is that they elaborate on complex situations without being limited by a highly structured form. A collection of anecdotal notes based on observable, factual performances can become the basis for justifying promotions and merit raises as well as suspensions and dismissals. If anecdotal notes are written immediately after a critical performance event occurs, the nurse leader's memory is not dimmed by the passing of time. And according to Barbara J. Stevens, anecdotal notes are critical to the first step in most agencies' disciplinary procedures.[6] In short, when a supervisor gives an oral warning to an employee about improper performance, anecdotal notes must be made to document the time, date, and circumstances under which the oral warning was given. Consider the following example:

> Today, from 1:45 to 2:10 PM, I discussed Shirley Archway's frequent absences with her. Specifically, we discussed that she had reported absent three times during the past 4 weeks—March 11, 19, and 27. I warned her that I could not tolerate her absences because her failure to report for work has caused a hardship for the rest of the staff. I explained that I was giving her an oral warning. If she is absent again within the next 2 months, she will receive a written warning followed by a 3-day suspension from work. These policies appear on page 46 of the 1981 *Employee Handbook*. Shirley looked at my copy of the *Handbook* for about 5 minutes. She then said that she understood she was receiving an oral warning and could be suspended for 3 days if she reported absent only once during the next 2 months. Shirley refused to give any explanation for her absences this month.

The head nurse dated and signed this written communication before filing it for future reference.

LETTERS OF APPRECIATION, PRAISE, AND GOOD WILL

Experienced nurse leaders recognize letters of appreciation, praise, and good will as excellent instruments for conveying recognition and positive feedback to members of the nursing staff. In the organizational communication setting, these letters are messages that you *don't have to write* but that you *really ought to write*. They build morale and enhance employees' and colleagues' self-esteem by giving formal credit for participating in demanding projects or for achieving significant professional awards.

Well-written letters of appreciation, praise, and good will are specific, concise, and personal. Enough details of an employee's achievements are mentioned so that the receiver of the message knows that the sender does, indeed, appreciate his or her special accomplishments. The tone should be friendly, sincere, and personal, yet free from obvious flattery. Copies of letters expressing appreciation or thanks for a job well done are often placed in employees' personnel files as a further means of enhancing their self-esteem and promoting recognition of their accomplishments.

Although messages of praise do not always contain the word *congratulations*, the sender certainly wants to highlight the receiver's special achievements. The concise, you-oriented note that follows was sent by one university nurse educator to a colleague:

> Your thorough book review of Joyce's new edition of *Medical-Surgical Nursing* was a delight to read.

You analyzed the book's specific strengths and weaknesses in such a professional, painstaking manner that I knew the editors of the journal had selected the right person to review this revised edition of a classic nursing text.

Congratulations on a first-rate review!

Letters of praise and appreciation can be written directly to the person, as the preceding message illustrates. But they may also be sent to a third person, often the employee's immediate supervisor. The next letter explicitly praises a nurse's successful presentation of an inservice program, but it also builds good will by acknowledging the nurse manager's support of the project in giving the nurse on-duty time to prepare:

Last week, Mrs. Victoria Langham presented four inservice programs to the nursing staff on the nurse's role in audiological testing. We in the staff development department were very pleased with her presentation.

With minimal assistance, Vicky determined the objectives and content of her program, composed a pretest and a posttest to measure the nurses' comprehension of the material presented, and demonstrated via the lecture-discussion format her knowledge of the subject. What is most impressive about Vicky's performance is that this is the first time she has taught in a classroom setting.

Thank you for giving Vicky on-duty time to prepare the inservice sessions.

Finally, some letters do *more* than express appreciation, praise, or good will. This last letter thanks the reader for promptly sending valuable information, and it also shares experiences and ideas with nursing colleagues:

Thank you for sending the description of your hospital's mobile float unit. It was good of you to get me the information so soon.

The mobile unit concept you describe has given us insight into how we might develop a permanent float unit at our institution. Upgrading the "traditional float pool" to a well-defined mobile unit, with its own head nurse manager, could improve the morale of our nursing personnel who are currently assigned to the float pool.

If we decide to implement a mobile unit, we'll send you the guidelines we draft.

SUMMARY

Nurses in leadership positions must frequently write requests justifying new equipment, increased staffing, or additional space. Justification reports may appear in memo or letter format, using either the direct approach or the indirect approach. The strategy for the direct approach (used when little resistance is anticipated) involves directly stating the request and then following it with a supporting explanation. On the other hand, the writer who chooses the indirect approach delays the request until late in the message, only after first arousing the reader's interest and then developing the rationale for the forthcoming request.

Proposals are persuasive reports that attempt to gain authorization for a specific and significant course of action. They may be classified according to audience, length and complexity, degree of formality, and whether they are solicited or unsolicited. Memo format is appropriate for informal internal proposals of three or fewer pages. For longer proposals, a modified report format with six headings is used. Main topic headings are introduction, process or methodology, management of tasks or objectives, financial considerations, personnel qualifications, and conclusions. Longer proposals may also include a title page, a table of contents, and an abstract.

A job description is a written summary of the relationships, responsibilities, and duties that compose a given position within an organization. Each job description helps implement the health care organization's philosophy, purpose, and objectives. Since it provides a framework for describing the performance elements of any job, its use is essential in developing a meaningful performance appraisal tool.

Components of the job description are department, job title, date, job summary, responsibilities, and job specifications. The critical performance components of the job description should be comprehensible to people both within and outside the nursing department. They should be specific enough so that people understand what they are to do, yet flexible enough to cover logically related (but unforeseen) job responsibilities.

Nurse leaders frequently participate in the performance appraisal process, which consists of three key elements: (1) the written evaluation based on objective work standards, (2) the feedback interview, and (3) the goal-planning session between the superior and the employee. The actual writing that the nurse leader does in documenting the performance review depends on the agency's performance appraisal tool, its performance review policies, and the degree to which the employee meets the job standards.

The most meaningful performance appraisal tools are those that use critical performance standards from the appropriate job description to help identify the categories in which the employee will be evaluated. Performance standards are identifiable, measurable achievement criteria that signify a level or baseline against which to measure an action or event.

Like behavioral or performance objectives, performance standards focus on performance—on what the employee does, produces, or achieves. Each standard begins with a specific and carefully selected action verb related to each critical performance activity.

Anecdotal notes can be used to document a variety of objective descriptions about an employee's performance. Usually, anecdotal notes are recorded in narrative form on plain paper, clearly stating who performed the specific behavior, who observed that behavior or event, and the time, date, and place that it occurred. Such messages should be timed, dated, and signed.

Letters of appreciation, praise, and good will are excellent instruments for conveying recognition and positive feedback to members of the nursing staff. Such letters are best written in a specific, concise, and personal style.

EXERCISES

1. Your nurse manager has approved the cardiac rehabilitation unit's request for two additional electronic infusion pumps. However, she needs a justification memo from you to make the request "official" when she presents the specialty nursing division's budget to the comptroller. Draft a justification report for the two infusion pumps to the nurse manager, using the direct approach. Remember that while your nurse manager does not need to be persuaded of the validity of your request, the financial committee will carefully scrutinize your arguments to see if your request is, indeed, justified.

2. Draft an informal proposal to the director of staff development, suggesting that your facility institute an orientation module on dealing with death and dying. Give the rationale for including the topic in the orientation program, with suggestions on how the content of the module should be developed and taught. Also, state the benefits that will accrue to the orienting nurses as well as to the agency.

3. Write a proposal of about seven pages on developing a group hypertension screening program in your agency's outpatient clinic. Follow the headings and format suggestions given in the text for proposals over four pages long.

4. If you are now employed in a health care facility, write down your current job description, applying the guidelines given in the text. How closely does this job description match the agency's written job description for your position?

5. Write a job description for the position you expect to have 5 years from the time you will complete your formal nursing education.

6. Analyze your agency's performance appraisal tool. Then write a short report of about 1,000 words on its strengths and weaknesses. Consider not only how well the performance standards are defined for each functional component of the job but also the appropriateness of the rating scale.

7. Examine both your agency's job description for a specific position (such as staff nurse) and its associated performance appraisal tool. Then write a 500-word report that explains to what extent the appraisal tool and job description correlate.

8. Review in the text the six performance standards for a primary nurse under the category of "Directing and Coordinating Others." Then develop and write about five or six performance standards for each of the *other* job components of a primary nurse, from assessing through making decisions.

9. Write clear, meaningful anecdotal notes for each of the following situations:

   a. You are the clinical nurse preceptor for a new graduate nurse who has been in orientation for 2 weeks on your busy surgical unit. Write four entries in your new graduate's record to demonstrate the progress the nurse has shown in initiating and maintaining intravenous infusions. Remember to document specific, observable behaviors and to date and sign each entry.

   b. You are the assistant head nurse on 8-East, a general medical unit. During the past week, you have noticed that whenever you ask Mrs. Johnson, a nurse's aide, to answer lights, pick up dietary trays, or take used supplies to central service, she always gets another aide to do what you have asked her to do. When you question Mrs. Johnson about this, she responds: "Well, someone else volunteered to do it for me."

   c. You witness a conversation at the nurses' station between Dr. Kilgarin and Nancy Richards, one of your team leaders. When Dr. Kilgarin becomes verbally abusive because the lab report for the partial thromboplastin time (PTT) isn't on the chart, Nancy calmly explains why. Dr. Kilgarin pays no attention to Nancy at first, but then she takes the physician aside into your office and confronts him assertively about his behavior. She handles the situation well, and you believe that Nancy's behavior demonstrates tact and sensitive interpersonal skills.

   d. Ann Jones, an L.P.N. team member on your unit, shows excellent judgment during a bomb-threat phone call. Document her performance in detail, explaining how she was able to keep the speaker on the line until the call was traced.

10. Write a three-paragraph letter of appreciation to Chris Locker for logging in many overtime hours in the clinic while beginning work on a master's degree. Chris's willingness to continue working full time until you found the right replacement enabled you to hire the best person to fill the position as nurse practitioner in the rheumatology clinic.

REFERENCES

1. Ann Brockenshire and Mary Jane O'Hara Hattstaedt, "Revising Job Descriptions: A Consensus Approach," *Supervisor Nurse,* 11 (March 1980), 16.
2. Brockenshire and Hattstaedt, p. 18.
3. Linda Pohlman Haar and Judith Rohan Hicks, "Performance Appraisal: Derivation of Effective Assessment Tools," *Journal of Nursing Administration,* 6 (September 1976), 24.
4. Susan Albrecht, "Reappraisal of Conventional Performance Appraisal Systems," *Journal of Nursing Administration,* 2 (March–April 1972), 31.
5. Ann Marriner, "Evaluation of Personnel," *Supervisor Nurse,* 7 (May 1976), 37.
6. Barbara J. Stevens, "Performance Appraisal: What the Nurse Executive Expects From It," *Journal of Nursing Administration,* 6 (October 1976), 29.

FURTHER READING

Cicatiello, Julian S. "The Personal Development Interview." *Supervisor Nurse,* 6 (November 1975), 15–24.

DeBakey, Lois. "The Persuasive Proposal." In *The Practical Craft: Readings for Business and Technical Writers.* Eds. W. Keats Sparrow and Donald H. Cunningham. Boston: Houghton Mifflin, 1978, pp. 208–227.

Partridge, Rebecca. "Evaluating Performance of Nursing Personnel." *Nursing Leadership,* 2 (September 1979), 18–22.

Rieder, George A. "Performance Review—A Mixed Bag." *Harvard Business Review,* 51 (July–August 1973), 61–67.

CHAPTER VI

Communicating Through Nonwritten Modes

Objectives

After studying this chapter, you will be able to

1. List the factors that influence the content of the intershift report.
2. State the purposes of the nursing report as a communication tool.
3. Distinguish among direction-centered reports, feedback reports, and intershift reports.
4. Summarize the advantages and disadvantages of conference reports and taped reports.
5. Discuss five points that will help ensure more meaningful taped reports.
6. Define the characteristics of effective listening.
7. Explain the barriers that can affect the rate of listening comprehension.
8. State the purposes of silence and its relationship to listening.
9. Describe eight measures to increase listening comprehension.
10. Define the scope of nonverbal communication.
11. Analyze the relationship between nonverbal communication and speech communication.
12. Summarize the influence of ethnicity on nonverbal communication
13. Discuss the array of messages conveyed by the face and the eyes.
14. Evaluate the use of the *mask* in professional nursing practice.
15. Analyze the nonverbal cues of posture and clothing and their influence on how professional colleagues and the public perceive the nurse's role.

In the first chapter, we introduced the concept that communication is a process largely dependent on adaptation. Indeed, the theoretical foundation for this book is that adaptation is the key to effective communication and to the entire communication process. A person's ability to send and receive many different types of messages and to adapt his or her sensory modalities and intellect to cope with them forms the basis of effective communication.

In this chapter on communicating through nonwritten modes, we focus on the adaptation process as it relates to the oral and nonverbal exchanges that nurses enter into during their day-to-day professional activities. Although the emphasis in this book has been on written communication, there is no doubt that the channels of speech, hearing, and observation are quite important to professional nurses in helping them communicate purposefully. To be sure, written *and* oral messages are essential to nurses who must report on their clients to the care givers who follow them. And yet the ability of nurses to listen carefully and to interpret nonverbal messages wisely *also* counts for a great deal when working with clients as well as nursing colleagues.

This chapter, then, concisely reviews the nature of report conferences, some concepts and skills of effective listening, and the essentials of nonverbal communication.

REPORT CONFERENCES

Most nurses participate regularly in report conferences. As primary nurses or team leaders, they give report to nurses who will be caring for clients after they (the reporters) leave the health care facility. And if they work with or manage auxiliary nursing personnel, they may also conduct direction-giving reports as well as feedback reports.

Because nurses work in a number of health care situations with a variety of client needs and problems, it is virtually impossible to establish a single set of criteria for reporting client information. The reporting mechanism must be guided by many factors, including the nursing department's philosophy of reporting, the agency's staffing pattern and ratio of professional nurses to ancillary care givers, and the type of clients cared for.

Although most acute care agencies have change-of-shift reports between the on-coming and the off-going nursing personnel, some agencies operate quite successfully without the formal, nurse-to-nurse intershift report. In extended care facilities, the report may be very brief if the client population is stable and there are few changes in the clients' nursing needs. Nurses working for public health agencies as primary care givers usually do not report on their assigned clients unless they are going on vacation or need to reassign clients to another care giver.

No matter what their content, all reports require purposeful, planned presentation. As a communication tool, reports should help care givers transmit relevant information, in a formal or informal setting, that enables nurses to formulate, modify, or revise the clients' nursing diagnoses and to evaluate plans of nursing care. Reports should aid nurses in organizing and prioritizing client care and in distributing client care assignments according to nursing care needs and nursing personnel's job classifications. In short, the oral reporting session can help nurses carry out assignments correctly and confidently.

We may summarize the purposes of nursing reports as follows:

- To communicate data relevant to the condition of clients
- To communicate progress (or the lack of it) to other nurses who will work with the clients

- To promote intershift communication and group participation in determining clients' nursing care needs
- To plan nursing care for individual clients and groups of clients
- To formulate, verify, or modify long- and short-term goals and nursing interventions based on initial nursing assessments
- To identify client problems and employ the problem-solving strategies of the nursing process in seeking solutions
- To evaluate the plans of nursing care for clients

Nurses in most agencies routinely use three kinds of reports: (1) direction-centered reports, (2) feedback reports, and (3) intershift reports. To learn about other types of reports (such as nursing rounds and case presentations), consult the list of further readings at the end of the chapter.

Direction-centered Reports

Direction-centered reports are conducted by the nurse leader after listening to the intershift report given by the off-going nurse and then making rounds to assess clients' health status. In other words, based on the nursing judgments of the previous nurse and on clients' input, the nurse leader is able to delegate specific nursing actions to the auxiliary nursing staff. Direction-giving reports—in fact, all oral reports and report conferences—should be held in a quiet conference room away from the distractions of the busy nursing unit. The nurse leader gives pertinent information about each client's care, such as diet and fluid status, diagnostic tests, and hygiene needs. Semistructured forms can be used to allow care givers to more quickly write down necessary information. If the unit secretary can transcribe these routine items, care givers can spend less time writing and more time listening.

The specificity of the directions the nurse transmits to the care givers depends on their job classifications, responsibilities, usual level of job performance, ability to grasp information, and type of clients cared for. Professional nurses cannot expect ancillary nursing personnel to respond correctly to the general direction: "Restrict Mrs. Reep's fluid intake." Although the message is brief, it tells nothing about the exact quantity, type, or timing of the fluid restriction. The professional nurse, of course, can quickly determine the amount of restriction based on the client's nursing and medical diagnoses and on a knowledge of the relationship between the client's physiological status and the principles of fluid balance. But unless the information is expressed specifically or concretely for auxiliary employees, they will be confused.

The nurse can also expect to spend more time giving specific instructions when new or complex nursing care activities are delegated to auxiliary employees, even if these activities are within the realm of their job descriptions. For example, if the L.P.N. has never applied plastic skin barriers in the treatment of decubitus ulcers, the registered nurse should anticipate spending extra time explaining the procedure as well as observing the L.P.N. when the dressing is applied.

Although direction-centered reports are often considered routine conferences for getting organized, the nurse leader conducting them must be sure that the directions are heard and understood. So that personnel can begin their work without unnecessary delay, the report should be brief. However, the nurse must guard against blocking feedback from care givers in an attempt to save time.

Feedback Reports

Since direction-centered reports essentially involve the downward flow of information from professional nurse to auxiliary personnel, the nurse must close the communication loop by holding feedback report sessions with the staff. Many agencies have such sessions about 1 hour before the workday ends. Certainly, active listening emerges as the most important tool that the nurse uses at feedback sessions. If the nurse does not listen to staff members' observations about their clients, they may lose interest, contribute nothing, and attend the sessions only because they have to.

Moreover, the nurse leader has to listen actively at feedback sessions to overcome the feeling that "I know what's going on." Indeed, the nurse has had many opportunities for receiving feedback to the direction-giving report during the workday by observing care givers complete their assignments and by assessing and interacting with clients. But only formal feedback reports, no matter how brief they must be, can provide both the nurse leader and the other care givers with a sense of completion. The data and observations that the auxiliary care givers report supply input to help the professional nurse revise and update nursing care plans, plan or modify the next day's client assignments, and organize the intershift report.

Intershift Reports

Nurses use intershift reports to inform on-coming nurses of changes in clients' conditions, therapeutic regimens, and nursing care needs. It is with intershift reports that the greatest variety occurs with the format and type of information communicated to nurses on the next shift. This variety stems from those organizational factors previously mentioned: the agency's philosophy, the individual nursing unit's philosophy, the communication and management expectations of the head nurse, staffing patterns, the size of the unit, and the type of clients and their nursing care needs.

The intershift report can be implemented via the traditional face-to-face conference between the on-coming nurse and the off-going nurse. Ancillary nursing personnel may or may not be present, depending on clients' conditions, staffing patterns, and immediate nursing care needs. Other ways of conducting intershift reports include taped reports and walking rounds. The latter method involves the on-coming and off-going shift nurses assessing each client's status at the bedside. In walking rounds, clients can become active participants in the intershift report; nurses talk *with* them, not *to* them or *about* them.

In her 1975 *Journal of Nursing Administration* article, Patricia M. Joy describes an intriguing modification of walking rounds that omits the formal nurse-to-nurse report at the bedside. Instead, the on-coming nurse makes rounds by communicating with each client. The client, then, becomes the main source of the on-coming nurse's report, supplemented with pertinent information from the Cardex, care plan, and chart. If the on-coming nurse needs to clarify information obtained from the client or from documentation, he or she can do so by talking with the off-going shift nurse.[1]

Although walking rounds and Joy's client-centered rounds are workable in many situations, the face-to-face report and the taped report remain the most popular vehicles for giving intershift report. And although agencies have used taped reports for several years, it is not uncommon for nurses to express a strong preference for the face-to-face conference report over the taped report. Proponents of face-to-face reports state that there are more opportunities for meaningful feedback—a chance to ask questions, clarify information, and directly share ideas about client care. Taped reports, according to these nurses, tend to relate information but with little mention of how the reporting nurse adapted or modified client care as a result of the information.

On the other hand, taped reports can be an effective communication tool for busy nursing units. When used properly, they can actually promote intershift feedback. Advocates of taped reports claim that they save time by omitting exchanges of information extraneous to client care. Planning before reporting is essential for all types of reports, but it is crucial when the report is taped, for there are no nonverbal cues to maintain the listener's attention when pauses in the recording occur. When the nurse who reports plans and organizes the information *first* before taping, the report can be concise and logical; it can also be a good summary of clients' conditions and can provide important nursing directives to maintain the continuity of care.

Are there certain situations when oral reports might communicate better than taped reports? It appears so. Marion Mitchell's survey of taped and oral intershift reports shows that nurses in specialty and critical care units prefer oral reports. These nurses claimed that the face-to-face exchange helps them have greater empathy with clients and view them more holistically. The efficiency, effectiveness, and conciseness of taped reports made little impression on the nurses surveyed. Clearly, the intershift collaborative and problem-solving process is an integral function of these nurses' oral reports.[2]

Nevertheless, apart from specialty and critical care units, taped reports can be effective and efficient, while incorporating feedback elements. The following five guidelines can help you give a more meaningful taped report:

1. Take several minutes to plan your report before you tape. Organize your notes from the report you heard when you came on duty, from your feedback conference, and from your client rounds. Determine what progress your clients made and what on-coming nurses need to do to continue the plan of care.

2. Coordinate your notes with the clients' care plans. You want to avoid just relaying information. And so, to make information meaningful for the nurses who follow you, put it within the framework of the nursing process and clients' individual plans of care.

3. Evaluate the amount of information you need to transmit to the next shift, the time frame, and the client care priorities. On units where there is a 30-minute shift overlap, keep the taped report to under 20 minutes so that nurses will be able to ask you questions before you leave. Although you will probably give your report in a sequential manner, according to the arrangements of a module or team, consider whether you can give it according to those clients with the most pressing or highest priority nursing needs treated first. Organizing your report according to clients and their needs, rather than geographical location, may help on-coming nurses better plan their workday. But whether you report according to room number or according to clients with the highest priority of nursing needs, finish your report on one client before going on to the next.

4. Play back the tape after reporting on the first client, to check for indistinct speech, garbled words, incomplete thoughts, or too slow or too rapid speech. Ask another nurse to evaluate the taped message for these flaws. Concentrate on giving clear, specific instructions whenever members of the next shift must complete a test or procedure begun on your shift.

5. Solicit feedback from members of the on-coming shift about the quality of your taped report. Ask to be told what was not clear and what

could have been omitted. Also, what helpful information should you have added?

EFFECTIVE LISTENING

The need to apply effective listening skills in all client care situations cannot be overemphasized. Much has been written about the nurse's purposeful listening in therapeutic client interactions. But sensitive listening practices are essential for all members of the health agency if the organization is to achieve its objective of delivering quality client-centered care.

When health care employees do not listen to the client effectively, displaying an attitude of concern and interest, care plans may be formulated inappropriately (perhaps because the nurse has listened with only "half an ear" when formulating the plan with the client or family), inadequate or unnecessary pain relievers may be given, and client diagnostic tests may be delayed. Ineffective listening can disrupt the relationship between client and nurse, nurse and nursing colleagues, among many others. Indeed, poor listening skills can cost the health agency thousands of dollars each year.

Of course, good listening skills are necessary for all daily activities, not only those involving direct and indirect nursing care in a health agency. Unfortunately, most people do not listen very well since they have not acquired, through formal or informal education, the prerequisite aural skills that lead to effective listening comprehension. As Ralph G. Nichols notes, most of us communicate verbally for about 70% of our waking hours, and of our time spent in verbal communication, about half (45%) is spent listening. As for the other verbal communication activities, 30% is spent speaking, 16% reading, and 9% writing.[3] Most schools, however, spend the bulk of their instructional time teaching reading and writing.

And perhaps because most of us have never been taught good listening skills and have not had the opportunity to develop increased aural comprehension, we may operate at only a 25% to 50% level of efficiency when listening to a 10-minute talk. In one experiment, students tested *immediately* after a 10-minute presentation demonstrated the ability to recall 50% of the material. When they were tested again *after 2 weeks,* their recall ability had decreased to 25%.[4]

An interesting parallel to the concept that we receive and attend to only 25% of the total verbal stimuli that we hear is illustrated in a 1975 research study that investigated what nurses communicated in a simulated change-of-shift report. After nurses listened to a series of tape-recorded vignettes giving specific information about a client with a particular health problem, they then reported to the next nurse about 25% of what they had heard. They did not give their reports solely on the information obtained; rather, they interpreted the information and gave specific nursing orders on how to manage the client's care.[5] In essence, this situation is typical of the types of reports nurses give each other. It also emphasizes the role of interpretation, which may impede or enhance effective listening.

How, then, do we define effective listening? Listening occurs *"when a human organism receives data aurally."*[6] But more than just receiving data, for effective listening to occur, the receiver must decode the data, then process it by comprehending and sharing the sender's meaning of the message. Effective listening is even characterized by certain physiological changes—the heart rate increases and the body temperature rises slightly.[7]

Barriers to Effective Listening

Why is it difficult for the average person to achieve a listening comprehension rate higher than 25% to 50%? Clearly, the main barrier is the rate of our "thought-speech" processes; in other words, we think at a much faster rate than we talk. Although we speak at the rate of 125 words per minute, thoughts race through our brains about four times as fast. Furthermore, physiologically it would be impossible for us to hear every sound that surrounds us, for the central nervous system would literally become bombarded by external physical stimuli. For the brain to make sense out of all the stimuli, much of it must be discarded in order for the meaning of the other stimuli to be perceived, interpreted, and reacted to. "As human beings," points out Dominick A. Barbara in *The Art of Listening, "our limit of absolute attention is only a few seconds*. We like variety and are easily distracted. . . . When we do not listen with real attention or interest, the information at hand seems monotonous and boring."[8]

The importance of effective listening in helping to complete the communication feedback loop should not be underestimated, either. When we listen poorly, we are unable to "play back" the sender's message. In the absence of relevant "playback," the feedback loop cannot close and the communication process is interrupted and disturbed—perhaps for seconds or minutes, perhaps for hours. Internal and external noise in the channel can hamper one's ability to listen effectively and greatly increase the chances for miscommunication. A variety of external stimuli can cause noise for nurses who suddenly have many demands to meet, but often our own internal noise, caused by our rapid thought processes, creates the greatest barrier.

Besides the rapid rate of our "thought-speech" processes, there are many other barriers to effective listening. In busy nursing units or outpatient facilities, nurses may not listen well because of sensory overload. Frequently, they receive too many demanding stimuli at once to process and attend to. The nurse who is told to give a preoperative medication an hour ahead of schedule to one client while listening to another client's disclosure about being afraid to die may be unable to listen effectively to one of the messages. And yet both are surely important. The ability to cope with competing messages is something that nurses must develop if they are to listen and communicate successfully in the health care setting.

Our own attitudes, biases, and preconceptions constitute another barrier to effective listening. We prefer to hear messages that support our own ideas because they protect our self-concept and our ideological self-worth. For example, nurses who value and support primary nursing will not be as open, in general, to listening to the administrator who supports functional nursing for cost containment purposes.

Being "mentally prepared" to hear one type of message and then having to receive another kind of message may be a very serious barrier to effective listening, especially in client teaching or counseling sessions. Consider the effective listening potential of the client who had surgery 6 days ago and is now prepared to go home, based on the discussion her physician held with her preoperatively. This client will not be likely to attend to the surgeon's rationale for her staying in the hospital a few days longer, even though she states that she is unhappy that she is not progressing at the rate she and other health care members had expected. In this case, the client's awareness of her status does not enhance her ability to hear a different message. The client had *expected* to hear that she could go home, and when she learned that she could not, she "tuned out" the message.

Listening and Silence

Down through the ages, silence has signified wisdom and intelligence, the foremost indicator that a person is being listened to when he or she seeks advice and counsel from a superior, colleague, or friend. But to human beings today, the relationship between listening and silence is often a frightening one, especially to those who believe that silence represents negative moods—anger, fear, rejection, or nonacceptance. To these people, silence becomes the primary means of communication with which they feel comfortable in expressing displeasure and anger. In psychotherapy and other therapeutic communication situations, however, silence can provide a sense of catharsis, especially after a particularly intense interaction.[9] And silence can be joyous, as Claudio states in Act II, scene i, of Shakespeare's *Much Ado About Nothing:* "Silence is the perfectest heralt of joy; I were but little happy, if I could say how much!"

Silence is the best tool at your disposal to help you develop good listening skills. The use of silence after listening to the sender's message, or after a particularly intense interaction, promotes closure of the feedback loop. Silence helps the listener decode the message and play it back to the sender. Or it can help the sender reflect on what he has said, providing him with the means to generate internal feedback and possibly clarify the message.

As a professional nurse, it is essential that you cultivate good listening comprehension skills in therapeutic client interactions. The success of your therapeutic use of self depends on your ability to accurately listen to and perceptively "tune in" on the client's message. But you also need good listening skills in your interactions with nursing colleagues, auxiliary nursing personnel, ancillary departments, and physicians. Indeed, the very delivery of client-centered care and its successful continuity depend on nursing professionals who demonstrate good listening skills in report conferences, interdisciplinary conferences, and staff teaching conferences. Since the average person's listening comprehension varies from 25% to 50%, it seems obvious that *not* listening, or becoming too relaxed about listening, will inevitably contribute to miscommunication.

Characteristics of a Good Listener

What are the characteristics of a good listener? And what can you do to improve your listening skills? The following eight points succinctly summarize the qualities of a good listener and give successful strategies for helping you to become a better listener.

1. You need to develop a genuine interest in and a humanistic concern for others. When you are genuinely interested in other people, you just naturally seem to listen better, perhaps because you have developed a sense of "interested commitment" in others. You need to resist the temptation to interrupt, to give advice, or to interject your own experiences. Hearing the speaker out may make you momentarily anxious, especially when you have a strong desire to help another. But your willingness to listen without interruption can greatly help the speaker's problem-solving ability. According to Ruth Strebe, "a good listener is one who facilitates the speaker's ability to solve his own problems and to grow interpersonally through greater self-understanding."[10]

2. You need to have an innate curiosity about the world and constantly ask yourself what potential relevance a seemingly dull topic can have

for you. Obviously, you won't listen as well to topics that don't interest you. So to increase your listening ability, try to determine how the topic can help you in your daily activities. Or ask yourself what connection there is between any subtopics and your own areas of interest.

3. You need to make an active, conscious effort to tune in auditory stimuli while filtering out noise and distractions. Sometimes the only way to filter out distractions is to physically move away from them. For example, if you give or receive report at a busy nurses' station, you will probably find it more difficult to listen to the person giving the report if the phone rings frequently and other nursing and ancillary personnel are using the client records. In this case, it would be far better to move to the conference room, where the report could be interrupted for emergencies by a communication system consisting of telephone, intercom, and emergency call signals. At other times, you may need to work diligently to filter out distractions (such as the client's television, the staff's discussion of a popular movie, and general background conversation) while you try to focus on visitors' questions.

4. You need to be aware of and respond to both the content and the affective component of the message. Often this affective level is not readily apparent in the content nor through such paralinguistic features as rate, tone, or presence of pauses. But when you ignore the message's affective component, you reduce your ability to project concern and interest. So take advantage of nonverbal cues such as eye contact, posture, gestures, and facial expression to help decipher the feeling tone of the message.

5. You need to listen for the purpose, main ideas, or essential points in every interaction. Facts are beneficial only as they support or hinder the effectiveness of the message. Whether you are listening to a co-worker's presentation on nursing implications of diabetic urine testing at a teaching conference or listening to a colleague's progress report on the feasibility of establishing a hospice unit, you will be more successful at remembering factual information if you listen for the main ideas or framework of the message. Facts can then be more easily integrated, and so remembered, since you can relate them to the main points.

6. As the active listener in the communication process, you need to give evidence of your involvement by providing the sender with feedback about how the message has been interpreted. You can do this by periodically *reviewing* or *summarizing* the information that the speaker gives you. *Restating* the message in your own words helps you express the speaker's intent, especially when he or she is unsure of the purpose of the message. *Reflecting* (or playing back) the message to the sender helps him or her clarify the message and make it understandable.

7. You should take notes as you need to while you listen. But be flexible. Successful listeners realize that there is no single note-taking system that is appropriate for all interactions.

8. You should use your spare thinking time to the best advantage. Your spare thinking time is the difference between thought-speech (600 words per minute) and the rate of speaking (125 words per minute). To use that time effectively, you can try to determine in which direction the speaker is heading, periodically review the main points, evaluate the speaker's evidence in support of the main points or thesis, and listen between the lines for pertinent nonverbal communication cues.[11]

NONVERBAL COMMUNICATION

Because of the dynamic relationship between verbal and nonverbal communication, it has often been said that you cannot *not* communicate. Every action, indeed every nonaction, has the potential to become the focus of a communication event. Communication encompasses all the modes of behavior that a person uses consciously or unconsciously, purposefully or without purpose, premeditatively or haphazardly, to affect the behavior of another human being. Indeed, the human communication process begins at birth with the infant's cry and stops at death with the cessation of the heartbeat.

The essence of nonverbal communication, then, is the symbolic, behavioral nonspeech event. Nonverbal communication has probably become one of the most truly interdisciplinary fields of all the social sciences; it has been strongly influenced by linguistics, anthropology, sociology, ethnology, psychology, and social psychology. The label *nonverbal communication* has been applied to "everything from facial expression and gesture to fashion and status symbol, from dance and drama to music and mime, from the flow of affect to the flow of traffic, from the territoriality of animals to the protocol of diplomats, from extrasensory perception to analog computers, and from the rhetoric of violence to the rhetoric of topless dancers."[12] For one authority, the transmission of one element—feeling—is the crucial identifying agent of nonverbal communication.[13] Other authorities have identified from 3 to 18 potential areas of nonverbal communication, including environment, machines, and pictures.[14]

Essentially, you can consider nonverbal communication as consisting of all those elements of nonspeech communication that transmit information and feeling in a conscious or unconscious manner. Usually, experts in the field of nonverbal communication cite three main areas: *kinesics,* the study of bodily movement and gestures; *proxemics,* the study of human beings' relationship to the organization of space; and *paralanguage,* those extralinguistic elements such as pitch, tone, and rate of speech that exist alongside the formal language structure.

As the transfer and exchange of information and feelings through such nonlinguistic modes as physical activities, gestures, facial expressions, touch, use of space, and paralanguage, nonverbal communication has several significant aspects. Most important of all is the notion that nonverbal communication is *not* an isolated or separate communication system from speech communication. Ray L. Birdwhistell, an anthropologist who pioneered the study of kinesics (or body language), argues that individual elements of nonverbal communication cannot be understood unless they are interpreted within the framework of the communication event. Anthropologist Edward T. Hall agrees with Birdwhistell, emphasizing the interdependence of the nonverbal message and the context of the spoken message: "Nonverbal communications must always be read *in context;* in fact, they are often a prominent part of the context in which the verbal part of the message is set. Context never has a specific meaning. Yet the meaning of a communication is always dependent upon the context."[15] In other words, neither speech communication nor nonverbal communication can relay the complete meaning of what a person is saying. Only when they are both considered and interpreted *together* do we have a good chance of understanding the message. And because our nonverbal cues operate on such a basic feeling level, it is often more difficult to control those activities. Perhaps that is why we tend to believe the nonverbal message instead of the verbal message when there is a conflict between the two.

In any kind of face-to-face interaction, probably our greatest tendency is to try to comprehend and react to what another person is saying. But if we concentrate only on what is said, we will probably not be successful receivers. Birdwhistell believes that about 65% to 70% of the meaning of any interaction is tied to associated nonverbal activities.[16] The realization that spoken words are responsible for only one-third of the meaning of the message is an awesome one. Obviously, being unaware of nonverbal communication cues could have a significant impact on your ability to successfully understand another's message.

Experts in the field of nonverbal communication agree that nonverbal systems are closely related to one's culture since messages can hope to be understood only within their cultural context. According to Birdwhistell, there are no gestures or actions that are universal symbols for all cultures.[17] Recent research indicates that certain facial expressions are universal,[18] but the general notion of nonverbal cultural dissonance is still widely held. That is, the chances of being able to accurately interpret nonverbal messages decrease as the cultural differences increase.[19]

Trying to decipher the elements of a culture's nonverbal communication system can be frustrating for health care workers, whether or not they are fairly fluent in the culture's language. This difficulty occurs basically because the nonverbal communication system in other cultures is much more extensive than our own. Furthermore, although most cultures or ethnic groups have a well-developed, highly structured linguistic system formally taught to most members of the cultural group, nonverbal communication is not systematically taught. So actually, when you learn a foreign language, you learn only one part of it—the formal structure of the verbal system. Albert Mehrabian emphasizes that there is "no systematic effort in this culture, or in most cultures, to try to teach a child how to express his feelings nonverbally. Considering this point, it is indeed very puzzling that there is any such thing as nonverbal communication."[20]

We will continue our discussion of nonverbal communication by touching on kinesics, the study of body language. For those who would like to know more about this area of nonverbal communication, as well as paralanguage, proxemics, territoriality, touch, and time, we suggest consulting some of the references at the end of the chapter.

Kinesics

In his *Body Language,* author Julius Fast popularized the study of what has become one of the most important and well-known elements of nonverbal communication—kinesics. According to Birdwhistell, kinesics is the "systematic study of how human beings communicate through language and gestures."[21] He divides the body into eight basic areas of kinesic activity: (1) total head, (2) face, (3) trunk and shoulders, (4) shoulder, arm, and wrist, (5) hand and finger, (6) hip, upper leg, lower leg, and ankle, (7) foot, and (8) neck.[22] Impressed by how closely kinesic activity was related to the linguistic structure of speech communication, Birdwhistell used the term *kine* to represent the most basic movement of any bodily activity. Thus, a wink is one of several kines related to eye movement. Classes or units incorporating related kines Birdwhistell called *kinemes.* Interestingly, he has identified 32 kinemes specifically related to activities of the face and head.

Closely related to the concept of kinesics are gestures, synchronized body movements that most members of an ethnic group agree have some specific meaning. They should be able to be "immediately interpreted" by the sender or the receiver of the message.[23] The research that Birdwhistell conducted in comparing the American to the English body movement system convinced him that gestures "not only do not stand alone as behavioral isolates, but they do not have explicit and invariable meanings." Like the stem forms in language, gestures require additional body cues to give them meaning in each interaction.[24]

The use of gestures varies according to gender, ethnicity, stress level, formal education, profession, and socioeconomic status. For example, it is widely accepted in this country that when students give a formal oral presentation, they are to control their use of gestures. In fact, the more formal the social situation, the more closely a person will control his or her body language, most probably the hands. In informal social settings, however, a person uses gestures and body language more freely to punctuate and emphasize the feeling tone of the message. Yet in some cultures, most notably the Italian and the Latin American, free use of body language is appropriate for almost all social situations. Birdwhistell memorably describes just how closely gestures are associated with language. When he viewed films, with the sound off, of former Mayor of New York, Fiorello LaGuardia, Birdwhistell was able to tell immediately when the politician was switching from English to Italian to Yiddish, just from his use of gestures![25]

Probably what is most striking in any discussion of kinesics is that body movement is essential for effective communication. Since up to 70% of the meaning of any message is conveyed by kinesics and other nonverbal cues, ignoring these cues could contribute to the distortion and misinterpretation of the message. The use of body language also helps us communicate those feelings and emotions that might be difficult to verbalize. You have probably seen many people who control their use of body language during formal situations, only to relax later with a less rigid posture or a freer use of shoulder, hand, and leg movement. John W. Keltner points out that whenever we can use the body to assist in communication, "we are rewarded by a release of energy and an increasing freedom of expression which apparently cannot be achieved by any other means."[26]

THE FACIAL DIMENSION

Of all the nonverbal modes of communicating, it is the face that is the most complex and the most capable of expressing an incredible array of emotions. Physiologists tell us that the muscles of the forehead, eyebrows, lids, pupils, nose, mouth, cheeks, and even ears can combine geometrically to give us thousands of unique facial expressions. The universality of facial expressions has long been a controversial topic, possibly because social scientists have been aware that gestures can be unique to one particular culture or have completely different meanings in other cultures. And so arose the assumption that facial expressions could not be universal.

Interestingly enough, just as Darwin argued over 100 years ago that basic facial expressions have universal meaning, so Paul Ekman's research supports this notion today. His study shows that the great majority of college students from five different cultures could agree on the meaning of six emotions (happiness, fear, surprise, anger, disgust/contempt, sadness) represented in selected pictures. Further research with isolated New Guineans (who had had very limited contact with Westerners) confirmed their ability to also identify the six facial expressions. So, Ekman's research seems to strongly suggest that the six facial expressions just cited do carry universal meaning.[27]

Usually, facial features move in harmony and in synchrony to reflect emotions such as fear, happiness, anger, or disgust. The more intense the message, the easier it is to interpret the message. But at times the face becomes hard to read. There are many reasons why this happens. The intensity of the emotion may have considerably diminished. Or one part of the face, such as the mouth, may show one expression, while another part, such as the eyebrows, shows another expression. Or expressions may move across the face so quickly, sometimes in as little as one-fifth of a second, that it becomes difficult for the casual observer to note them. Yet these *microfacials* often occur when people try to hide their feelings.[28]

At other times our faces become masks, either displaying a blank expression or substituting for the emotion we really feel one that is more socially acceptable or more in harmony with our own self-concept. The teenager who fears having blood drawn every few hours may wear the mask of anger whenever the nurse draws his blood. Although anger is not usually considered a socially acceptable emotion, it may be more acceptable to the teenager in preserving his self-concept than admitting his fear of "needles."

Many situations exist that demand that we intensify, deintensify, neutralize, or mask our expressions. In some segments of middle class American society, widows are expected to assume the "grieving but coping" mask for the funeral. This mask permits the widow to be sorrowful, but it discourages crying and sobbing—or any other overt expression of mourning. But the widow who comes from an ethnic group that values vocal expressions of mourning could not wear the "grieving but coping" mask without being considered cold and lacking emotion. Wearing that mask might even eventually cause her to become socially isolated from her family and community support group, just when she most needs their psychological support.

Without a doubt, most nurses wear a professional mask at some time during their careers. Until recently, nurses have usually worn a mask when dealing with other health care workers, most notably physicians. Nurses often mask their feelings in caring for clients with disfigurements, malodorous fistulas, or draining decubitus ulcers. Sometimes the mask is put on when working with clients who have a particular problem or diagnosis. One of our colleagues once confessed that she was consciously aware of putting on a mask every time she worked with clients who had had myocardial infarctions. "It took a lot of soul searching," she added, "until I realized that I could not be an effective care giver or teacher—that I could not even build trust!—until I took off my mask."

In one view, the professional mask of a nursing supervisor is an "oblong toothy smile . . . accompanied by expressionless eyes."[29] In wearing a mask with a smile, we choose well, believes Julius Fast, "for a smile is a sign not only of humor or pleasure but it is also an apology, a sign of defense or even an excuse."[30]

Although the professional mask may help the nurse overcome a particularly stressful event, wearing it constantly, especially in interactions with clients, only decreases the nurse's therapeutic use of self. Sidney Jourard implies that when nurses consistently mask their expressions as a result of their educational background and clinical experiences, they develop a "character armor"—"a case of rigid interpersonal behavior."[31] The problem with the professional mask, then, is that it may become transformed into an inauthentic, emotionless behavior pattern that can be extremely harmful to the nurse-client relationship.

EYES AND EYE CONTACT

In discussing the part that the face plays in the study of kinesics, we cannot overlook the significance of the eyes. Eyes have long been considered the physiological entrance to a person's spirit, soul, or uniqueness. The nineteenth century Spanish novelist and essayist Miguel de Unamuno once wrote: *"Los ojos son las ventanas del alma"* ("The eyes are the windows of the soul"). As the organs of sight, the eyes by themselves do little to deserve this acclaim. The emotions that the eyes discharge are related to the face's accessory organs of sight—lids, lashes, brows, and periorbital skinfolds.

A person's eyes can strike up a variety of poses, such as wide-open eyes to express amazement and squinty eyes to convey skepticism, but the most significant factor in the eyes' ability to communicate is eye contact. For example, we avoid eye contact with others when we feel uncomfortable or if we do not want to take time to talk. If we avoid eye contact while we are still talking, it may mean that we are clarifying our thoughts and that we wish to avoid interruptions from the listener.[32] Once we turn our gaze back, however, and lock gazes with the listener, we send out the signal that it is permissible to interrupt us when we pause.[33] In other words, we are ready to receive feedback.

People who make limited eye contact when they speak usually manage to convey a lack of interest or concern in the listener. They diminish the sense of trust that they may have previously established or else harm the chances of building it at this time. Obviously, direct eye contact promotes the trust relationship. The significance of eye contact is so great, in fact, that deaf persons rely on it heavily to supplement their conversation in sign language.[34]

The amount of eye contact in any given social interaction also seems to be highly dependent on a person's ethnicity. A 1970 cross-cultural study of the variables affecting human behavior in relation to the arrangement of space showed that Arabs (especially Egyptians) and Latin Americans use the most eye contact during interactions, whereas Americans use the least.[35]

Another intriguing aspect of eye contact is what sociologist Erving Goffman calls *civil inattention*. As we walk down the street, through a busy corridor, or in any public place, our eyes pass over the eyes of others, but without pausing with a look of recognition. Goffman says that we permit ourselves to "eye" each other until we are about 8 feet apart. After that, each person lowers his or her eyes until the other passes—a phenomenon Goffman calls "a kind of dimming of the lights."[36]

Appearance

People can also send out a powerful nonverbal message by means of their appearance—posture, clothing, hairstyle, make-up, and jewelry. Briefly, we will discuss the nonverbal cues of two of these aspects—posture and clothing—and the implications of the messages they transmit in the health care delivery system.

POSTURE AS A NONVERBAL CUE

People's posture, that is, the degree of physiological tension that affects how they walk, sit, or stand, is an important source of nonverbal communication. The cues that they transmit are frequently read to determine status or position, degree of self-confidence and self-worth, and liveliness or fatigue. The message that people with slumped shoulders send is far different from the one that people send who stand erect, hold their shoulders back, and make good eye contact. The first message might be read as fatigue, apathy, depression, or laziness. The second indicates alertness, readiness for action, interest, or discipline.

Our body posture is even a good indication of how much we respect (or even fear) those with whom we come into contact. The young graduate nurse may experience a few imperceptible changes in posture when she talks to the head nurse about routine expected changes in client needs. But during the performance appraisal process, the new nurse may feel more tense, and her posture will probably reflect this increased tension. She may not sit completely back in the chair. Her shoulders will probably be straight, her head erect, and her legs uncrossed (or crossed only at the ankles), with both knees together. Mehrabian cites a similar example of a change in posture that occurred with a young dentist. His body language changed noticeably when his older, distinguished partner spoke to him: "He moved forward in his seat, leaned forward, moved his knees together, and clasped his hands."[37]

CLOTHING AS A NONVERBAL CUE

The clothing that people wear can also convey a powerful nonverbal message. Along with the dress that people choose to wear, accessories to appearance—such as hairstyle, use of scent, and such artifacts as jewelry, glasses, or hearing aids—help define their body image as well as reflect to some degree their self-concept. In general, clothing can suggest people's socioeconomic status, mood or emotional status, sense of fashion, and profession or work roles.

Perhaps no item of clothing conveys more about people's professional and/or work roles than a uniform. Sociologist Goffman suggests that police officers, as well as nurses, are "open" people—people that the public need not have an excuse to approach for information or advice. What makes nurses "open" people is largely a function of the uniform they wear.[38] The uniform gives the public tacit permission to ask the person who wears it for help, advice, or comfort.

The uniform can also help employees within an agency, as well as the public, more readily identify others in various work or professional roles. In large agencies, the uniform can even simplify the communication network when personnel from different ancillary service departments dress in different styles or colors of uniforms. So the uniform identifies the person's role and function in the agency and even sets up guidelines for potential interactions.

The uniform or type of clothing that the nurse wears may determine how his or her role is defined. So strong is the symbolic identification of the white uniform and cap with the role of the nurse that it often becomes difficult for the public, as well as an agency's nonnursing administration, to admit that nurses need not wear white to be nurses. Historically, white has symbolized purity, goodness, and exemplary conduct. Yet it can also represent authority, aloofness, and coldness. Many people's fears of health agencies and health care workers can be traced to childhood experiences when they were "surrounded by people in white uniforms" before an especially stressful procedure. To avoid fostering the association between the nurse dressed in white and discomfort or illness, many pediatric units encourage their nurses to wear colored or printed uniforms. Nurses working in acute care psychiatric units wear street clothes instead of uniforms to minimize the association by clients, family, and even other nursing and ancillary personnel of clients' maladaptive coping mechanisms signifying emotional disorders with the medical model of mental illness based on disease pathology.

Nurses can also transmit subtle but significant messages about their status or role when they wear lab coats over uniforms or street clothes. In some agencies where nurses routinely wear white uniforms, wearing a lab coat over a uniform may consciously or unconsciously indicate a higher, supervisory status. When a new group of affiliating students came to one hospital to begin their clinical experience, several of them thought, erroneously, that all nursing supervisors wore lab coats. (The day that the students met the supervisors, all were wearing lab coats, quite by chance.) Later on, the students had difficulty trying to determine just who was a supervisor, since laboratory technicians occasionally wore lab coats over their uniforms, too.

Another message that the lab coat over street clothes conveys is one of increasing independence in nursing practice or increased managerial responsibility. To the staff nurse who wears a white uniform, the street clothes and lab coat that the clinical nurse specialist or nurse practitioner wears can indicate that these practitioners are responsible for delivering direct care to individuals or groups while still having time to teach, consult, or do research. Perhaps the message is: "I'm a nurse, but I'm in a different, more specialized role." Head nurses who need to emphasize to the staff their managerial role and related administrative responsibilities find that wearing street clothes and a lab coat can convey that message very well.

Just as clothes play an important part in the nurse's nonverbal message system, so are they an important source of nonverbal messages for the client. Clients who wear agency gowns or robes transmit the message that they are having diagnostic tests or that they do not have their own clothes with them. We have observed that some clients prefer institutional gowns to their own night clothes, even when there is no chance of damaging them or soiling them. Although we know of no systematic research done on the topic of why clients would prefer the agency gown to their own, it could be that such a choice reflects a conscious or unconscious desire to transmit the message: "I'm so sick I should wear a hospital gown." As most nurses know, often the first indication that clients are feeling better, both physiologically and emotionally, is the decision to wear their own clothes, shave or put on make-up, and fix their hair.

SUMMARY

Professional nurses use the nonwritten channels of speech, hearing, and observation to enable them to make clear, concise intershift reports, to listen effectively to clients and colleagues, and to interpret nonverbal messages wisely.

Most nurses usually participate on a regular basis in reporting conferences. The type of report they give is guided by the philosophy of the nursing department, the agency's staffing pattern, the ratio of professional nurses to ancillary care givers, and the nursing care needs of the clients. Purposes of the report include to communicate clients' conditions, their progress, and priorities of care; to identify problems and formulate goals and nursing interventions; and to evaluate care plans.

Direction-centered reports, feedback reports, and intershift reports are three types of communicative reporting tools that nurses often use. The modes of making intershift reports include face-to-face presentations, walking rounds, and taped messages.

The ability to develop sensitive listening skills is essential for ensuring the communication feedback loop in collegial relationships as well as in therapeutic nurse-client interactions.

Effective listening occurs when the receiver attends to aural data and shares the sender's meaning of the message. Because most people's thoughts race along at 600 words per minute (though they are able to speak only one-fourth as fast), people often set up their own internal barriers to keep them from listening effectively. Our listening comprehension rate usually averages only 25%.

In addition to the internal noise of rapid thought-speech, other barriers to effective listening are external channel noise; sensory overload (or receiving too many messages at one time to attend to them); our beliefs, attitudes, and values; and messages contrary to what we expect to hear.

Silence, an important adjunct to listening, helps close the feedback loop by letting the receiver play back the message to the sender. Or it can provide the sender with time to reflect on the message, in effect enabling him or her to generate appropriate internal feedback.

People can improve their listening skills by being genuinely interested in others, developing a natural curiosity about the world, filtering out distractions while tuning in on auditory stimuli, and being aware of both the content and the process of the message. Listening for the purpose of the message helps make factual information more relevant, as does using a flexible note-taking system. Most importantly, making use of spare thinking time helps the receiver evaluate the speaker's ideas while listening between the lines for significant nonverbal communication cues.

Nonverbal communication consists of all those elements of nonspeech communication that transmit information and feeling in a conscious or an unconscious manner. Frequently cited components of nonverbal communication are kinesics, the study of bodily movement and gestures; proxemics, the study of human beings' relationship to the organization of space; and paralanguage, those extralinguistic elements such as pitch,

tone, and rate of speech that exist alongside the formal language structure.

Nonverbal communication is not a separate, isolated system from
speech communication. It can be understood and interpreted only when it
is considered within the entire context of the message. But because nonverbal behaviors are less easily controlled, when there is a discrepancy
between the verbal and nonverbal messages, we are more inclined to believe the nonverbal cues. In this sense, nonverbal communication can be
considered a human lie detector.

Since messages must be interpreted within the cultural framework, the
greater the cultural disparity between the communicators, the less likely
they will be able to interpret nonverbal messages accurately. Gestures,
synchronized symbolic movements, may be unique to one ethnic group; or
they may have different meanings in different cultures.

Of the eight areas of basic kinesic activity, the face and head are most
capable of expressing a wide array of emotions. Recent research indicates
that six facial expressions are universal to all cultures. Sometimes the
actual lack of genuine facial expression becomes the expression. This is
known as the *mask*.

The accessory features of the eye—forehead, brows, lids, and periorbital skin folds—contribute heavily to the eyes' expressiveness. Although
the eyes can strike up a variety of poses, the most significant factor in the
eyes' ability to communicate is eye contact.

Posture and clothing are two other elements of nonverbal communication that transmit powerful messages. The uniforms, lab coats, or street
clothes that nurses wear can convey significant messages about their
roles.

EXERCISES

1. Role play a 5- to 10-minute reporting session with another student or
    colleague. Base your presentation on four to six clients you have cared
    for in your recent clinical experience. Have other members of the class
    record and evaluate your nonverbal behavior, including eye contact,
    gestures, and the proportion of time you spend talking, listening, and
    writing. Also ask them to record and evaluate the manner in which
    you provide verbal and nonverbal feedback. If you have access to video-
    tape equipment, record the session. Then, follow it up with a written
    report on the tape that analyzes both nurses' listening skills and non-
    verbal behavior.
2. Your clinical nursing coordinator strongly supports the idea of elimi-
    nating the formal intershift report on the 36-bed orthopedic unit

where you work as a team leader. You were not in favor of the concept when you first heard the coordinator discuss it; but after talking with her several times, researching the topic, and seeing the advantages, you believe it is worth trying as a pilot project for 60 days. The rest of the unit doesn't share your view but believes instead that the disappearance of the formal intershift report can only contribute to the deterioration of the unit's communication system. The coordinator has asked for your help in trying to "sell" the idea to the staff. You agree to do so by using the following strategies:

a. First, research the topic by reviewing the current literature on intershift reports. Patricia M. Joy's article, cited in the references, is a good place to begin.

b. Next, prepare a two-page proposal for the unit personnel, using persuasive strategies that will help to convince them to adopt the project on a trial basis.

c. Finally, defend the proposal orally to the members of the class (who will role play the reluctant, doubting members of the unit).

In writing your proposal and in preparing your oral defense, you should anticipate being able to address the following points of concern to the unit personnel:

- How they will find out what happened to the client during the day if there is no formal report
- When the project will begin
- How the project will be implemented
- The mechanism to evaluate how successful the project is
- How to ensure clients' continuity of care
- How to use the shift overlap time effectively

3. Give a 10-minute oral report analyzing the notes from other colleagues or students who all attended the same lecture or class meeting. What sorts of variation do you see in their systems of taking notes? As you gather and organize the data, consider the following items:

- Format
- Use of drawings, pictures, or diagrams
- Type of note paper
- Use of abbreviations—standard and nonstandard
- Identification of main points
- Ratio of single words and phrases to complete sentences
- Length of notes

4. Analyze the notes you have taken in at least four *different* classes or lectures. Do you see evidence of having changed your system of note

taking to meet each speaker's mode of delivery and message? If so, explain.

5. Prepare a 2,000-word written report on how personal space and territoriality (as elements of nonverbal communication) affect the nurse's delivery of client care in a busy ambulatory care facility. As a point of departure, you will want to consult Edward T. Hall's book, *The Hidden Dimension,* which gives a model for the organization of four interpersonal distance zones. Articles by Minckley, Pluckhan, Sommer, and Stillman (complete references are included in the Further Reading section) should also prove helpful, as should the first few chapters of Robert Ardrey's book, *The Territorial Imperative.*

REFERENCES

1. Patricia M. Joy, "Maintaining Continuity of Care During Shift Change," *Journal of Nursing Administration,* 5 (November–December 1975), 28–29.
2. Marion Mitchell, "Inter-Shift Reports—To Tape or Not to Tape," *Supervisor Nurse,* 7 (October 1976), 38–39.
3. Ralph G. Nichols, "Do We Know How to Listen? Practical Helps in a Modern Age," *The Speech Teacher,* 10 (1961), 118.
4. Nichols, p. 120.
5. Kenneth A. Wallston and Barbara S. Wallston, "Nurses' Decisions to Listen to Patients," *Nursing Research,* 24 (January–February 1975), 21.
6. Carl H. Weaver, *Human Listening: Processes and Behavior* (Indianapolis: Bobbs-Merrill, 1972), p. 5.
7. Nichols, p. 122.
8. Dominick A. Barbara, *The Art of Listening* (Springfield, IL: Charles C Thomas, 1958), p. 88.
9. Antonio J. Ferreira, "On Silence," *American Journal of Psychotherapy,* 18 (January 1964), 111.
10. Ruth Strebe, "Just What Do You Hear?" *Supervisor Nurse,* 2 (May 1971), 29.
11. Nichols, p. 124.
12. Randall P. Harrison and Mark L. Knapp, "Toward an Understanding of Nonverbal Communication Systems," *The Journal of Communication,* 22 (December 1972), 343.
13. Albert Mehrabian, *Silent Messages* (Belmont, CA: Wadsworth, 1971), p. 111.
14. Harrison and Knapp, p. 346.
15. Edward T. Hall, *Beyond Culture* (New York: Anchor Press, 1976), p. 70.
16. Ray L. Birdwhistell, *Kinesics and Context: Essays on Body Motion Communication* (Philadelphia: University of Pennsylvania Press, 1970), p. 158.
17. Birdwhistell, p. 81.

18. Paul Ekman, "The Universal Smile: Face Muscles Talk Every Language," *Psychology Today,* 9 (September 1975), 35–39.

19. Hall, p. 65.

20. Mehrabian, p. 111.

21. Ray L. Birdwhistell, "Background to Kinesics," *ETC: A Review of General Semantics,* 13 (Autumn 1955), 10.

22. Birdwhistell, *Kinesics and Context,* p. 258.

23. Birdwhistell, "Background to Kinesics," p. 16.

24. Birdwhistell, *Kinesics and Context,* p. 80.

25. Birdwhistell, *Kinesics and Context,* p. 102.

26. John W. Keltner, *Interpersonal Speech-Communication: Elements and Structures* (Belmont, CA: Wadsworth, 1970), p. 115.

27. Ekman, pp. 35–39.

28. Randall P. Harrison, *Beyond Words* (Englewood Cliffs, NJ: Prentice-Hall, 1974), p. 121.

29. A. Jann Davis, "Body Talk," *Supervisor Nurse,* 9 (June 1978), 36.

30. Julius Fast, *Body Language* (New York: Pocket Books, 1970), p. 54.

31. Sidney M. Jourard, *The Transparent Self,* 2d ed. (New York: Van Nostrand, 1971), p. 181.

32. Harrison, p. 126.

33. Fast, p. 141.

34. Mary Ritchie Key, *Paralanguage and Kinesics* (Metuchen, NJ: Scarecrow Press, 1975), p. 86.

35. O. Michael Watson, *Proxemic Behavior: A Cross-Cultural Study* (The Hague: Mouton, 1970), p. 77.

36. Erving Goffman, *Behavior in Public Places* (New York: Free Press, 1963), p. 84.

37. Mehrabian, p. 28.

38. Goffman, pp. 125–126.

FURTHER READING

Ardrey, Robert. *The Territorial Imperative.* New York: Atheneum Publishers, 1966.

Barnett, Kathryn. "A Theoretical Construct of the Concepts of Touch as They Relate to Nursing." *Nursing Research,* 21 (March–April 1972), 102–110.

Blondis, Marion N., and Barbara E. Jackson. *Nonverbal Communication With Patients: Back to the Human Touch.* New York: Wiley, 1977.

Bosmajian, Haig A. *The Rhetoric of Nonverbal Communication.* Glenview, IL: Scott, Foresman, 1971.

Cline, Victor B., Jon Atzet, and Elaine Holmes. "Assessing the Validity of Verbal and Nonverbal Cues in Accurately Judging Others." *Comparative Group Studies,* 3 (November 1972), 383–394.

Ekman, Paul, and Wallace V. Friesen. "Hand Movements," *The Journal of Communication,* 22 (December 1972), 353–374.

Georgopoulos, Basil S., and Josephine M. Sana. "Clinical Nursing Specialization and Intershift Report Behavior." *American Journal of Nursing,* 71 (March 1971), 538–545.

Haggerty, Virginia C. "Listening: An Experiment in Nursing." *Nursing Forum,* 10 (1971), 383–391.

Hall, Edward T. *The Hidden Dimension.* New York: Doubleday, 1966.

———. *The Silent Language.* New York: Doubleday, 1959.

Janz, Nancy, Agnes Buback, and Martha Simons. "How Shared Nursing Rounds Pay Off." *RN,* 40 (March 1977), 45–48.

Leathers, Dale G. *Nonverbal Communication Systems.* Boston: Allyn & Bacon, 1976.

McCorkle, Ruth. "Effects of Touch on Seriously Ill Patients." *Nursing Research,* 23 (March–April 1974), 125–132.

Meerlo, Joost A. M. *Unobtrusive Communication: Essays in Psycholinguistics.* Assen, The Netherlands: Van Gorcum Ltd., 1964.

Mehrabian, Albert. *Nonverbal Communication.* Chicago: Aldine-Atherton, 1972.

Mezzanotte, E. Jane. "Getting It Together for End-of-Shift Reports." *Nursing76,* 6 (April 1976), 21–22.

Minckley, Barbara Blake. "Space and Place in Patient Care." *American Journal of Nursing,* 68 (March 1968), 510–516.

Montagu, Ashley. *Touching: The Human Significance of the Skin.* New York: Columbia University Press, 1971.

Muller, Patricia A. "Using an Active Listening Model." *Supervisor Nurse,* 11 (April 1980), 44–45.

Nichols, Ralph G., and Leonard A. Stevens. "Listening to People." *Harvard Business Review,* 35 (September–October 1957), 85–92.

Okun, Sherman K. "How to Be a Better Listener." *Nation's Business,* 63 (August 1975), 59–62.

Pluckhan, Margaret L. *Human Communication: The Matrix of Nursing.* New York: McGraw-Hill, 1978.

———. "Professional Territoriality: A Problem Affecting the Delivery of Health Care." *Nursing Forum,* 11 (1972), 300–310.

———. "Space: The Silent Language. . . ." *Nursing Forum,* 7 (1968), 386–397.

Shapiro, Jeffrey G. "Variability and Usefulness of Facial and Body Cues." *Comparative Group Studies,* 3 (November 1972), 437–441.

Sommer, Robert. "The Distance for Comfortable Conversation: A Further Study." *Sociometry,* 25 (March 1962), 111–116.

———. "Leadership and Group Geography." *Sociometry,* 24 (March 1961), 99–110.

————. "Studies in Personal Space." *Sociometry,* 22 (September 1959), 247–260.

Stillman, Margot J. "Territoriality and Personal Space." *American Journal of Nursing,* 78 (October 1978), 1670–1672.

Summers, Ann. "Give Your Patient More Personal Space." *Nursing79,* 9 (September 1979), 56.

Unangst, Carol. "The Clinician's Use of Nursing Rounds." *American Journal of Nursing,* 71 (August 1971), 1566–1567.

Viscott, David. *The Language of Feelings.* New York: Arbor House, 1976.

CHAPTER VII

Researching and Writing for Publication

Objectives

After studying this chapter, you will be able to

1. Identify writing resources that enhance the nurse author's ability to make a commitment to a writing project.
2. Discuss factors that determine the appropriate topic on which to write.
3. Differentiate among the nursing indexes in conducting a review of the literature.
4. Explain the advantages of using computerized searches in conducting a review of the literature.
5. List factors that contribute to the journal selection process.
6. Discuss the purpose and characteristics of a query letter.
7. Analyze the process of planning, organizing, and outlining.
8. Evaluate the relationship between writing, rewriting, and revising.
9. State six guidelines to improve the use of language and style.
10. Summarize the steps in preparing and submitting a manuscript for publication.

Now more than ever, nurses are seriously engaged in writing for publication. They write book reviews for state nurse association journals; abstracts of current information for agency newsletters; letters to the editors of newspapers, lay journals, and professional journals; articles ranging from brief 500-word personal accounts to 5,000-word research reports; and full-length books. Staff nurses write on a variety of clinical experiences, from trying new approaches to nursing care to working with clients with complex needs. Master's-prepared clinical nurse specialists educated in research methodlogy write to report the results of their clinical studies. Nursing administrators write about new approaches to the management and delivery of care. And nurse educators write about their efforts to restructure curriculums, as well as about the results of their participation in educational and clinical research.

The reasons for the growing interest in writing for publication are varied, but many relate directly to nurses seeing nursing as a unique profession, one that is distinct from both medicine and the allied health professions. To communicate these differences to others and to inform the profession of the burgeoning knowledge base for the theory and practice of nursing, writing for publication becomes *the* communication vehicle. Thus, during the past 5 years, there has been an increase in the nursing literature in the number of articles and editorials on writing for publication. Writing workshops especially designed for nurses have also increased, thus reflecting an obvious interest on the part of nurses to refine their writing skills and to update their knowledge about how to get their ideas into print. And journal editors report an upsurge in the number of manuscripts to review for possible publication.

This chapter, then, will give a brief overview of the process of professional writing, specifically as it relates to writing articles for publication. We will discuss writing resources; topic selection; literature review; journal selection; planning, organizing, and outlining; writing, rewriting, and revising; and manuscript preparation and the editorial process.

WRITING RESOURCES

From previous chapters in this text and from your past experiences in writing, you are aware that writing for publication is a multifaceted process demanding the resources of time, environmental and psychological supports, and intense personal commitment. Because writing is a process that usually cannot be hurried, it is wise to do a careful self-analysis to determine whether you have the necessary intrinsic and extrinsic resources that can help you make the commitment to undertake a writing project.

First, consider the available time you have to write. And this means not only time to write but also time to plan, organize, and research your ideas, as well as integrate your thesis with the background materials you have researched. There is no way you can know how long a writing project "ought" to take. Timing is highly individualized, depending on your own natural flair for self-expression; your command of grammar, style, and language; your knowledge of the topic; and the amount of background research you need to do. But realize that the time you will actually need to complete a writing project will probably be at least twice as long as your first estimate.

Consider also whether you can handle the scope or the extent of the writing. Some writing projects are so broad in scope that it is difficult to "get a handle" on them. You also need to determine what your purpose or goal is in writing an article. For faculty members who must publish to secure tenure and promotion, the goal of writing is often just that—tenure and promotion. But there are many other goals and many other factors that might motivate you to write, such as the need to share important research, the desire to contribute to the advancement of nursing theory and practice, or the wish for recognition and accolades from colleagues, supervisors, and employers. Perhaps writing is a way for you to feel "self-actualized." The reasons are not as important as your awareness of what motivates you to write.

Finally, consider whether you have sufficient support—both environmental and psychological—to help you as you undertake a writing project. Some writers can work in the midst of numerous distractions, but most of us need the security of a quiet, private environment where we can work without interruption. It doesn't matter whether it's at the kitchen table or at a desk in the family room, as long as it's a place where you feel comfortable working. It's also best to pick a time of day when you're at your peak and to plan your writing activities during those hours. If your employer has asked you to write up a project at your institution to submit for publication, it's also important to negotiate work time for that activity. Too often, willing employees are eager to accept the challenge of writing, but they are left with insufficient resources (lack of time and/or an inadequate, distracting work environment) to accomplish the task. The eagerness quickly turns to disappointment and frustration as the employee realizes that he or she is unable to accomplish the project.

Because working on a writing project usually becomes an intensely personal experience, it is important to seek out people who will give you emotional and psychological support. Don't be swayed by those colleagues and acquaintances who are not interested in your writing or who say that you are foolish to spend so much time on a project that may never be published. Instead, cultivate the support and backing of those family members and friends who will encourage you in your efforts while helping you maintain a sense of humor.

With all the inner resources that you need to write, you may very well ask yourself, "Why even bother?" Aside from the contribution you may make to the body of nursing knowledge, and apart from the recognition you may receive from other professionals, writing can be a very growth-producing, satisfying experience. True, writing does not come easy to most people. And it can be painfully hard work. But there are few more challenging, more exciting activities to stretch the creative and intellectual horizons of the professional nurse.

TOPIC SELECTION

Once you have made the decision to write for publication, how do you decide what to write about? The most important consideration is to write about what you know. Just as the most successful modern novelists wrote about their families, communities, and unique experiences, so should you use what you already know or what you have already experienced as a foundation for your article. Or, if you discover serendipitously something that intrigues you, try writing on that topic. But you will need to be especially careful to thoroughly review the literature and take the time to integrate and synthesize your thoughts with the information you gain *before* you begin to write. Otherwise you might not have a good enough "handle" on the topic to convince the editor (and your audience) that you are qualified to write on the subject.

Not everything you know or find intriguing is the basis of a good, publishable article, however. You need to consider what your intended readers will find useful and how they can incorporate this knowledge into their nursing practice. Also, consider whether what you have learned or experienced will influence their attitudes or values, possibly helping them to see a new side to a formerly one-sided situation.

One writer suggests three broad categories of articles suitable for journals: current nursing problems, anticipated future roles, and health maintenance issues.[1] Other commentators identify five possible topics: the case study; the research article; articles on procedures, processes, and techniques; the historical article; and articles on current trends.[2]

Once you have selected your topic, narrowing it becomes crucial. Most general nursing journals accept articles between 1,500 and 4,000 words long. At 250 words per typed manuscript page, that amounts to 6 to 16 pages. Obviously, with this kind of restriction on length, broad or unfocused topics would not be suitable. Nor would the editors (or the readers they represent) find them interesting. Another reason to narrow the topic is so that you are better able to develop it and work with it. But you should be careful not to narrow it prematurely during the literature review. The subject of narrowing a topic is beyond the scope of this book, but you will find that the first two chapters of John Herum and D. W. Cummings's book, *Writing: Plans, Drafts, and Revisions,* give helpful advice on how to gradually narrow down and zero in on your topic.[3]

LITERATURE REVIEW

After selecting your topic but before you begin to narrow its scope, you will want to review the literature written in that area during the past few years. The exact number of years you decide to review will depend on what aspects of the topic you expect to deal with, as well as the depth and scope of the subject. Usually, it is helpful to review the literature of the past 5 to 10 years.

Many valuable library resources exist to help you review the literature for your chosen topic—the card catalog; indexes from nursing, medicine, and allied health; abstracts; directories; and on-line computer systems, to name just a few. A good place to get acquainted with the variety of library sources available for nursing is the July 1980 article in *Nursing Outlook* entitled "Reference Sources for Nursing."[4] Prepared by a committee of the Interagency Council on Library Resources for Nursing, the article supplies a current listing of abstract journals, bibliographies and book lists, dictionaries, drug lists, histories, and research and statistical sources, among others.

Another new reference that the nurse writer will find indispensable is the *Guide to Library Resources in Nursing* by Katina P. Strauch and Dorothy J. Brundage.[5] The first section opens with a description of general reference works, followed by an annotated listing of books and references in the major areas of nursing: medical-surgical nursing, the natural sciences, mental health and psychiatric nursing, education and nursing, administration and nursing, and research and nursing. Periodicals most appropriate to each area are listed at the end of each part. The second section gives a general introduction to the library, including detailed information on the methodology of conducting computerized library searches.

Indexes are probably the most valuable tools to help you research the literature efficiently. Most journals, including the *American Journal of Nursing, Nursing Outlook, Nursing,* and *Supervisor Nurse,* publish yearly indexes with the last issue. These can help you quickly locate an article, especially if you remember having seen it during the year or if you do not need to do a thorough, systematic search. But for broader-based searches, four indexes can be especially useful: the *Cumulative Index to Nursing & Allied Health Literature,* the *International Nursing Index,* the *Nursing Studies Index,* and the *Hospital Literature Index.* Because they are so useful, and because most small libraries have at least one of these indexes, we will discuss each one briefly.

The oldest nursing index, the *Cumulative Index to Nursing & Allied Health Literature* (CINAHL), was first published in 1956 by the Glendale Adventist Medical Center in Glendale, California. Before 1977, it was known as the *Cumulative Index to Nursing Literature.* There are five bimonthly issues yearly, with the annual bound volume appearing each March. CINAHL indexes over 200 English-language periodicals related to the fields of nursing, health education, and medical technology. In addition, it indexes all the American Nurses' Association's periodicals and pamphlets, all serials published by the National League for Nursing, and all the state nurses' associations' journals.

To use CINAHL efficiently, consult the "yellow pages" subject heading listing in the back of each annual volume. References are entered under both subject heading and author. Separate appendixes list book reviews, pamphlets, films, filmstrips, and recordings.

By far the index with the widest scope, the *International Nursing Index* (INI) has been issued quarterly since 1966 with an annual cumulation. Published by the American Journal of Nursing Company and the National League for Nursing in cooperation with the National Library of Medicine, INI compiles the listings of articles from over 200 international nursing journals, as well as nursing-related articles in over 2,000 non-nursing journals in the *Index Medicus,* the major medical index.

Like CINAHL, INI has separate subject and author sections to simplify the information retrieval process. It also features a listing of nurses' doctoral dissertations in the yearly volume. Foreign-language articles appear at the end of each subject heading, enclosed in brackets. The *Nursing Thesaurus,* appearing with the first yearly issue as well as in the annual cumulation, serves as a cross-reference index to correlate specific nursing topics with the Medical Subject Heading (MeSH) system used in both INI and the *Index Medicus.*

The annotated *Nursing Studies Index* is a retrospective compilation of nursing literature, including books as well as periodicals, from 1900 to 1959. Prepared under the direction of Virginia Henderson at Yale University, Volume I covers 1900–1929; Volume II covers 1930–1949; Volume III covers 1950–1956; and Volume IV covers 1957–1959. Extremely valuable for its historical approach to the development of clinical practice, nursing education, and nursing research, the *Nursing Studies Index* is the only index for the years 1900–1956.

Another index that nurses in managerial positions might consult is the *Hospital Literature Index,* an international subject-author index of English-language journals on health care administration. Published since 1945 by the American Hospital Association and since 1978 in cooperation with the National Library of Medicine, it is issued quarterly with annual cumulations.

Although you can usually find almost everything you need through the appropriate use of indexes, computerized searches can greatly ease the literature review, especially if the topic is complex and different aspects are listed under more than one index subject heading. The National Library of Medicine, located in Washington, D.C., provides several "on-line" information systems concerned with medical, nursing, and related health topics. With a data base of over 3,000 journals (including 250 in nursing), MEDLINE, or the MEDical Literature Analysis and Retrieval System on-LINE, can help locate quickly literature from the past 2 years on any specific biomedical subject in nursing, dentistry, medicine, or allied health. If you need information that goes back more than 2 years, MEDLARS can provide it from 1966. However, this search must be conducted "off-line," and the information must be mailed to you.

Other computer on-line information systems that the National Library of Medicine maintains include TOXLINE for citations to published human and animal toxicology studies, EPILEPSYLINE for references to epilepsy, and AVLINE for audiovisual materials in the health sciences. CANCERLIT provides 75,000 citations on all aspects of cancer; CANCERPROJ gives summaries of current international cancer research projects.

A number of large university and medical libraries in the United States have direct access to MEDLINE through their own computer terminals. With direct access, library patrons are able to gain access to the information they have requested in just a few minutes, either via computer print-out or cathode-ray screen. If the library does not have direct access to MEDLINE, it can still request the search through the appropriate Regional Medical Library. There is usually a small charge for computer searches, but most researchers believe that the cost is reasonable.

JOURNAL SELECTION

As you begin the process of selecting and narrowing your topic and reviewing the literature, you also need to identify the audience for whom you are writing. Elizabeth Kinzer O'Farrell's concern with audience identification and writing to meet reader needs is aptly addressed in her article, "Write for the Reader, He May Need to Know What You Have to Say."[6] In writing for publication, audience identification is virtually synonymous with selecting the right journal. So choose the journal with care. It may be the most important factor in getting your manuscript accepted for publication.

Review the journals critically for the past 2 years, even the ones you read regularly, to check the length, style, tone, and degree of formality of the articles. It's also a good idea to see how references are presented. Note the variety in the journal's format. Do all the articles seem to be written alike? Or are there stylistic differences from article to article? Are there special columns or features that might prove an appropriate vehicle for your topic? Are the articles well documented, with outside sources clearly indicated? Are there articles dealing with challenging client cases? If so, are they related to a specific category of nursing or type of client condition? How often are photographs, graphs, and illustrations used? In short, getting a feel for the types of articles that the journals present can help you identify the audience and so adapt your writing to meet the needs and interests of journal readers.

One recent survey of 65 English and foreign-language nursing journals can help you quickly compare the most pertinent characteristics related to the manuscript submission process. Although the data are not complete and some information may no longer be current, the survey is valuable for relaying important information for the nurse to be aware of when choosing where to submit a manuscript: the range of article word length, the number of copies to submit, the usual time needed to reach an editorial decision, the percentage of solicited and unsolicited manuscripts published, and the acceptance rate of unsolicited manuscripts.[7]

Discovering whether a publication accepts unsolicited manuscripts is an important aspect of the manuscript submission process. *Nursing Outlook* and *Geriatric Nursing* accept unsolicited manuscripts, but both advise that it is best "to query the editor in advance as to interest in the subject." Both the *American Journal of Nursing* and *Supervisor Nurse* state in their masthead that they accept original unsolicited manuscripts; they also add information about their manuscript requirements. On the other hand, *Nursing Clinics of North America* solicits almost all its articles, whereas the *Journal of School Health* publishes *only* unsolicited articles.

Once you decide on the most appropriate journal to submit your article to, you should write a letter of inquiry (a query letter) to the editor to see if the journal is interested in receiving a manuscript on your proposed topic. In fact, as just noted, *Nursing Outlook* and *Geriatric Nursing* recommend the query letter to prospective authors in their masthead. The purpose of the query letter is to help the author find out if the editor is interested in an article before he or she invests a great deal of time developing it into a finished product. Although you may get an encouraging reply to a query letter, the journal cannot promise to publish the article until it sees the finished product. Some authors and editors believe that you should not begin to write the article until you receive a positive response to your query letter. But we think that it is wise to have completed at least an outline or preliminary draft of the article. That way, when you query the journal, you can give the editors a realistic target date by which they might expect your completed manuscript. If too much time elapses between the date the query letter is received and the date the manuscript is submitted, editors may no longer be interested in the article. Or they may have decided to publish another manuscript that reached them sooner.

Query letters should be typed on quality white bond paper. They should be brief, certainly not over one page long. Address them to the editor of the journal. You can easily find out the name of the current editor from the masthead. Be sure to look at the most recent issue, however. There is nothing worse than writing to a person who has not been with the journal for the past 2 years. Such lack of attention to details shows the editor that you may be careless or hasty in preparing the manuscript.

The query letter should have a strong introductory or lead paragraph to arouse the editor's interest in your article. In effect, the query letter becomes a "sales letter," trying to convince the editor that you can write effectively and that your article will benefit the editorial scope of the journal. The letter should give the proposed manuscript's specifications: its length, how it differs from other similar articles, and the number of photographs or diagrams, if any, as well as why you are qualified to write on this topic. (Don't include a complete biographical résumé, however.)

And most importantly, you need to let the editor know when to expect the finished manuscript, once you have received a positive response to the query letter.

PLANNING, ORGANIZING, AND OUTLINING

Planning, organizing, and outlining your topic are essential steps in the development of an article for publication, as they are for any written project—proposal, report, term paper, or senior project. Omitting these activities or devoting insufficient time to them will make the actual writing phase much harder, if not impossible. You may become frustrated and confused, perhaps believing erroneously that you cannot write. In all likelihood, it is probably not that you cannot write but that you have not taken enough time to plan, organize, and outline what you want to write. As a nurse, you do not expect to give quality care without assessing clients and planning relevant goals and interventions. Nor should you, as a writer, expect to produce a topnotch article until you have assessed your journal audience's characteristics and planned the message to meet their needs. In general, the ratio of time spent in planning, organizing, and outlining to actual writing is 2:1. So, for every hour that you write, you should have spent 2 hours planning, organizing, and outlining how you were going to manage the task of writing.

Just exactly how does the writer go about organizing the ideas, thoughts, and background gleaned from the review of the literature? Organization should begin as soon as the library search starts. All types of aids can be used—index cards, separate notebooks, folders, even blank pieces of paper—as long as the writer develops a system.

Index cards are still the best means to record bibliographic information, ideas, direct quotations, and paraphrased information. The cards can easily be sorted later, according to their place in the outline. The 4" × 6" size seems to work better than the 3" × 5" because there is more space to record. When recording data on the cards, use the top line to note briefly in which category or section of the article the information belongs. If you are not sure, leave the top line blank so that you have space to add a title later. Brief titles can be indispensable in helping you sort and categorize the cards after you complete the library search.

Take care to make accurate notations when you record information on index cards; it will save you time in verifying incomplete references as you write the paper. Avoid using unusual or nonstandard abbreviations on the cards; you may not remember them later. For example, you may find yourself wondering if "NVCs" means "nonverbal communications" or "nonverbal cues." Only checking the source will clarify the situation.

Be sure to put quotation marks around direct quotations, indicating the page and the source at the bottom of the card. As long as you have a complete bibliographic reference to the source on another card, all you need put on the bottom of the note card is the author's name and page number: Stevens, p. 63. If you have two or more sources written by the same author, you need to include the name of the source: Stevens, *First-Line Patient Care Management*, p. 70.

Record complete bibliographic information for books and journals on title cards. Many writers who do extensive research, often using two or more libraries, write the call number on the title card as well as the library where they obtained the book. If they need to see the resource again, having the call number saves them time. (Saving the back copy of interlibrary loan requests is a good idea, too. If you need the book later on, the information on the back copy speeds the request.)

Folders can also be useful for sorting and organizing copies of journal articles. Writing the complete bibliographic data on the first page of the article can be a real timesaver later, as you organize your sources. Usually, most of this information is already on the first page or two of the copy. All you need to do is add the volume number or month and year.

Making an outline of your article is another essential step in the planning and organizing (or prewriting) process. Outlines are never "carved in stone"; they are modified to some degree during the research and planning phase. Think of them as guidelines to good writing, for they force you to plan and organize your thoughts logically, cohesively, and coherently. They also help you break up the writing into manageable pieces so that the process doesn't seem so overwhelming.

Probably the biggest concern that many beginning writers have is when to outline. Actually, you should do two types of outlines: a preliminary one to guide you in your search of the literature, and a revised, more detailed working outline after your complete the research and begin to define seriously the scope of your article. The preliminary outline may be nothing more than three main points, with perhaps two or three subheadings. It does not matter whether you use the decimal system or the number-letter system of outlining. Both help you accomplish the goal of outlining, namely, the planned, purposeful organization of thoughts and ideas to achieve a desired message. A preliminary outline, then, might look like one of those at the top of page 263.

As you prepare your working outline, you will probably change the order of the main points and subheadings. You may even discard one or two to replace them with more salient headings that you have determined from your research. As you continue, you add an introduction (with a strong lead paragraph), a summary, and more detailed subheadings. It is also a wise idea to define the article's purpose or goal (often referred to as a thesis statement) after the introduction, so that you don't

```
1.                    I.
   1.1                   A.
   1.2                   B.
2.                    II.
   2.1                   A.
   2.2                   B.
   2.3                   C.
3.                    III.
   3.1                   A.
   3.2                   B.
```

lose sight of what you want to accomplish. Writing each main point on a separate piece of paper is a good idea when outlining, for then there is more space for you to develop in greater detail the points you wish to cover.

A working outline, then, might be diagrammed like one of these:

```
Introduction            Introduction
Thesis statement        Thesis statement

1.                      I.
   1.1                     A.
   1.2                     B.
      1.21                    1.
      1.22                    2.
2.                      II.
   2.1                     A.
      2.11                    1.
      2.12                    2.
   2.2                     B.
   2.3                     C.
3.                      III.
   3.1                     A.
   3.2                     B.
      3.21                    1.
      3.22                    2.
         3.221                  a.
         3.222                  b.
   3.3                     C.
Summary                 Summary
```

If you should have a hard time getting started or difficulty organizing your ideas into a workable outline, you might try the brainstorming technique. Some writers report that combining brainstorming with outlining gives them good results. Brainstorming fosters creativity and the free flow of ideas; outlining enhances organization, molding the ideas into a logical sequence.

The purpose of brainstorming is to get many thoughts and ideas down on paper so that relationships among them can be recognized and used. When you brainstorm, you forget about whether ideas are good or bad, clearly phrased or poorly written. The task is simply to get as many ideas as possible down on paper. Then, after the brainstorming session, you can organize related concepts and outline the topic in a logical, sequential fashion, omitting any irrelevant ideas.

WRITING, REWRITING, AND REVISING

As we have said before, writing is a dynamic process. So after you write a first draft of your article, you will probably need to revise and rewrite that draft (or parts of it) several times. But if you do a thorough job of organizing and outlining your material, and if you take enough time to review the literature, narrow the topic, and synthesize your ideas with information you gather from the library search, writing will not be as difficult a task as you might have first expected.

When you do sit down to write the first draft, write it as quickly as possible. Don't worry at this point about grammar, spelling, or punctuation. Simply write! If the project is long, you might consider drafting the piece in sections. Then, once the draft is completed, put it away for at least a day or two before you begin to revise. This intermission will help you look at the draft with an analytical eye, an essential component of the rewriting phase.

During the time that you are revising and rewriting, you will need to look at three separate yet related aspects of your work: (1) logic, sequence, and order, (2) language and style, and (3) punctuation and spelling. It is only by systematically analyzing your own work in each of these areas that you will be assured of a quality manuscript.

Logic, Sequence, and Order

First, look at how the parts of your article fit together to form a whole. Then, look for inconsistencies in logic, sequence, and order. Do you have a good lead paragraph that arouses the reader's interest in your article? Does the introduction present the purpose or thesis of your writing? Do the main points show a logical sequence of development? Do the subtopics follow the main points naturally? If you have reached a conclusion, will your reader also be able to reach it without grasping for isolated pieces? Is your summary strong, an effective overview of what you have tried to present?

It is important to take sufficient time to analyze the merits of your lead paragraph or introduction. In Jane L. Binger's article, "Writing for Publication: A Survey of Nursing Journal Editors," introductions were often cited as not arousing the readers' interests.[8] The purpose of the lead paragraph is to attract the audience's attention, telling them briefly about the article by addressing the who, what, when, where, why, and how of the content. Just as the lead paragraph of the query letter must sell your writing potential to the journal editor, so also must the article's opening persuade busy professionals that *your* article will make interesting, worthwhile reading. You can get a good idea of different types of effective openings by analyzing those that capture your attention in various newspapers and magazines and in the journal to which you have chosen to submit your article.

During the revision phase, the "cut-and-paste" method can save you a lot of time in rewriting. If you decide that paragraphs are out of order, simply cut the manuscript and rearrange the sections to reflect the more logical sequence. Next, pay careful attention to the transitional phrases. As you read the draft of the manuscript, it may seem that paragraphs are out of sequence or that sentences are misplaced. Actually, what may have happened is that you omitted the statements or phrases necessary for making the logical transition from one point to another. Transitional phrases can show sequence, consequence, comparison, contrast, and time-space relationships. Typical transitional words and phrases are

- First (second, third, last)
- Consequently
- As a result
- Therefore
- For this reason
- Similarly
- By comparison
- On the other hand
- For example
- Later on
- The next hour (day, month, year)
- In short
- At the same time

Language and Style

After you are convinced that the article fits together well as a whole, you can begin second-stage revision for language and style. Depending on how "readable" your first draft is, it may be wise to rewrite the manuscript before attempting this revision process. Because most writers often make many changes in language and style, typing the second draft with triple spacing between each line will usually give plenty of room for needed revisions.

It is beyond the scope of this book to delve deeply into the intricacies of language and style. However, several good manuals of style are available—many of them delightful to read—that can help you improve and refine your writing technique. Among them are Strunk and White's *The Elements of Style*,[9] Barzun's *Simple and Direct: A Rhetoric for Writers*,[10] and Baker's *The Practical Stylist*.[11] Nevertheless, following these six brief guidelines can help you write more effectively by improving your use of language and style:

1. *Use natural language.* Natural language is not informal or colloquial language. Neither is it stilted or erudite. It *is* simple and direct. It sounds right. Binger's survey of editors from seven nursing journals cites the abuse of "overly formal writing" as a frequent weakness in authors' manuscripts.[12]

2. *Use jargon judiciously.* Like other professions, nursing has developed its own vocabulary to enhance communication. But professional terms can quickly become meaningless jargon when they no longer convey what they should.

3. *Avoid the passive voice.* Probably nothing weakens writing more than the liberal use of the passive voice. Consider the difference in impact between "Jack *was helped* every day with his dressing changes" and "Sarah helped Jack every day with his dressing changes." The first sentence illustrates the passive voice. It is weak compared with the second sentence. It is not at all clear who the agent was who helped Jack with his dressing. The second sentence uses the more dynamic active voice. It is clear who acted.

4. *Use qualifying words cautiously.* Words such as *very, somewhat, rather, basically,* and *little* can weaken style. And depending on elaborate adverbs and adjectives to strengthen your writing is usually false economy. They increase the wordiness of the material without increasing its forcefulness. Instead, select emphatic nouns and verbs to carry the thrust of the message.

5. *Make abstract concepts understandable.* The more theoretical your writing, the greater the need you will have to make it understandable

and readable for your audience. Examples, anecdotes, and case situations can make practical and concrete the abstract. Often, just two or three well-chosen examples will illustrate and clarify complicated information.

6. *Avoid gender-specific (stereotyped) language.* No singular pronouns exist in English that refer to *both* he and she, *both* his and hers. Used frequently, *he* or *she* and *his* or *hers* are awkward and burdensome for the reader. Many strategies exist for avoiding gender-specific language. Using the plural form of the noun to avoid a gender-specific pronoun is one solution: "All potential employees came to their interviews prepared to discuss goals and objectives." Another alternative is simply to omit the pronoun. Instead of saying "The empathetic nurse cares about her clients' feelings," you can drop the pronoun *her*: "The empathetic nurse cares about clients' feelings." For other examples of ways to avoid gender-specific language, see Shaffer and Pfeiffer's article, "Eliminate Stereotyped Writing."[13]

Punctuation and Spelling

During the third stage of the revision process, read the paper aloud, section by section. Reading aloud will help you not only check your progress in revising for style and language but also catch errors in spelling and punctuation. If you have not yet typed a draft, now would be a good time to do so. Typing helps you spot spelling and punctuation errors more readily. Be sure to use a standard college dictionary to check spelling. And consult an English handbook for questions on the correct use of punctuation.

MANUSCRIPT PREPARATION AND THE EDITORIAL PROCESS

Before you type the final copy of the manuscript for submission, check the masthead of the journal to see if there is any information for prospective authors. For example, *Supervisor Nurse* gives specifics on the number of copies to submit and on typing requirements. If the journal does not have this information on the masthead page, you can usually obtain it by requesting a copy of its manuscript guidelines.

However, several general guidelines apply to the manuscript format for most nursing journals. The article should be typed, double-spaced, on a machine using either elite or pica type. The typewriter should make clear, clean copy. Smeared type or imperfectly printed letters detract from the manuscript's appearance. Generous margins are necessary for the copy editing process, so they should be at least 1″ all around, except for the left-hand margin, which should be 1½″. Good-quality heavy bond paper is preferable to erasable paper, since the latter does not take corrections well.

Begin the manuscript by typing your name, address, telephone number, and place of employment or university affiliation in the upper left-hand corner of the first page. (Number the following pages consecutively in the upper right-hand corner, putting your name before each page number.) Then, go down five spaces and begin the article by centering the title. If the journal requires an abstract (a 35 to 100-word informative summary of the article), it may precede the title. Often, however, the abstract appears on a separate page, preceding the manuscript proper.

Use liquid paper correction fluid sparingly. If you find it necessary to make too many corrections or if you need to "white out" more than a word or two, consider retyping the page. Too many corrections can be distracting.

Proofread the manuscript *several* times before you send it, using at least two different means of checking for errors. No matter how carefully you have proofread the article, sharp editors will spot any typographical mistakes, misspelled words, and errors of omission of words or phrases. They stand out glaringly, distracting the editor and indicating rightly or wrongly that you have been careless in the preparation of the manuscript.

One way to proofread effectively is to use a red pen to circle the letters, words, and punctuation marks that need to be corrected on a duplicated copy of the manuscript. Red ink quickly identifies the errors, and using a duplicated copy prevents the original from being accidentally smeared or damaged during the proofing. Another method is to place a ruler under each line of the manuscript to focus your attention only on those words. The ruler forces the proofreader to read slowly and helps prevent the eyes from wandering over the rest of the page. Reading each word aloud also helps focus on the letters in the word, rather than on the word as a whole. Proofing the manuscript by reading it backwards can help, too, since you are not concentrating on content. Probably the best way to catch all errors is to ask two other people, besides you, to proofread the manuscript.

Take special pains to double-check direct quotations (are quotation marks properly placed directly before and after the citation?), footnotes, and bibliographic sources. Be certain to include accurate page numbers for your footnotes. Omitting them is one sure way to hinder your manuscript's acceptance or publication. You can get a good idea of the specific format to follow for references and footnotes by studying examples in past journal articles. Or the journal's manuscript guidelines will give specific instructions for documentation.

Follow the journal's guidelines for obtaining permission for the use of direct quotations. Some journals, such as *Nursing Outlook, American Journal of Nursing,* and *Geriatric Nursing,* permit the author to quote up to 500 words from any one issue without writing for permission. Other journals are more stringent. Probably it is a good rule of thumb to obtain permission for any quotation over 100 words.

Submit your manuscript with a cover letter addressed to the editor. Indicate briefly the subject of the article, along with your qualifications and background. If you received a positive response from a query letter, be sure to mention that, too. If the journal has asked for an abstract of the article when it is submitted, this may be included in the text of the manuscript (as already described). Or it may be typed on a separate piece of paper, following the cover letter.

Most editors advise sending the article by first-class mail so that it reaches the editorial offices promptly. Place the cover letter, abstract, original article, and required number of copies between pieces of sturdy cardboard in a large manila envelope. Do not fold the letter or manuscript. You should also enclose a self-addressed envelope with the correct postage attached, so that the manuscript can be returned, if necessary.

Most importantly, never send a copy of the article without sending the original. The editor may think that you are submitting the manuscript to another journal at the same time. Although it may be frustrating for the author to wait for the editor's reply, it is not proper to make multiple submissions of the manuscript. Editors have become very suspicious of this practice, and "they look with a jaundiced eye upon those writers who may have dispatched their Xeroxed copies to five different journals simultaneously."[14]

After the editor receives your article, you can usually expect to hear in 1 to 2 months whether your manuscript has been accepted for publication. The process may take longer, however, if the journal is refereed, because articles must then be read and critiqued by two or three editorial associates or consultants outside the journal's regular editorial staff. Even if the journal is not refereed, the decision process may take many months because of the large volume of articles that the editors receive.

If your manuscript is accepted, when can you expect to see it published? According to McCloskey's survey, it is not unusual to wait 6 months, or as long as 1 year, before the article is in print. The use of "article banks" (that is, earmarking accepted articles for inclusion in a series), the copy editing process, and the need for journals to make plans for future issues—all contribute to the delay. But once nurse authors see their work in print, they usually agree that the wait was worthwhile.

What if your manuscript is rejected? Read the letter of rejection carefully. It will probably give you some valuable clues, specifically mentioning one or more of these categories:

1. *Timing*. Your topic may not have been current. Perhaps too much has been written about it recently. (Did you do a thorough literature review?) Or, unknown to you, the journal may expect to publish a similar article in the near future.

2. *Audience*. If the letter says, "Your article is well written, but it doesn't meet our needs," you have not selected your audience and your journal with enough care. So try again! Remember that choosing the right journal is probably the single most important step in getting an article published.

3. *Writing*. If your organization or logic was faulty, if you neglected to include an attention-getting introduction and a strong summary, if you had overly turgid writing, your manuscript was probably rejected. Try again. Good writing is within your reach. Ask friends to critique your writing. And read well-written books and articles on a regular basis. Good writers read extensively. But they do more than just read. They analyze what makes some writing good and what makes other writing weak.

SUMMARY

During the past few years, more and more professional nurses have become actively involved in writing for publication. They write to share personal and professional experiences, to contribute to the expanding body of nursing knowledge, to obtain recognition for research efforts, to fulfill personal needs, and to achieve promotion in clinical and/or academic settings.

Writing for publication can be extremely rewarding. But it is also a demanding activity, requiring the resources of time and environmental and psychological supports. In addition, the potential author must usually make an intense personal commitment to the writing project.

Nurse authors greatly increase their opportunities to become successfully published when they write about topics with which they are familiar. Topics must usually be current, pertain to nursing practice, and deal with a concept, idea, or nursing intervention that other professionals can put into use in their area of nursing. Carefully defined, limited subjects are usually preferable to those that are more general in scope.

Many valuable resources are available to help nurse authors review the literature on their chosen topic: the card catalog; selected library guidebooks; a variety of nursing, medical, and allied health indexes; abstracts; directories; and computer systems. Four indexes are especially useful: the *Cumulative Index to Nursing & Allied Health Literature,* the *International Nursing Index,* the *Nursing Studies Index,* and the *Hospital*

Literature Index. MEDLINE, the National Library of Medicine's on-line computer information system, can quickly locate the most recent literature on any specific biomedical subject.

During the literature search is a good time for authors to carefully identify the audience for whom they wish to write. Journals print articles to meet the needs of their readers, often a fairly specialized group of professionals with associated specialized reading interests. So articles that do not meet the needs of a journal's readers will not be published. Selecting the appropriate journal may be the single most important element in getting a manuscript accepted for publication. Authors write query letters to journal editors before they submit completed manuscripts, to determine whether it is worthwhile to pursue the development and refinement of their articles.

Planning, organizing, and outlining are crucial steps to complete before writing the initial draft of the manuscript. Two types of outlines are useful in this prewriting phase. The preliminary outline guides writers in the literature search; the revised, more detailed outline becomes an essential tool to guide the development of the first draft.

After the first draft is completed, writers must revise their work for miscommunication in the following areas: (1) logic, sequence, and order; (2) language and style; and (3) punctuation and spelling. Errors in logic or sequence can often be corrected by the "cut-and-paste" method of rearranging paragraphs. Guidelines for achieving appropriate language and style include using natural language, eliminating unnecessary jargon, avoiding the passive voice, employing qualifying words cautiously, using concrete examples to make the abstract understandable, and avoiding stereotyped language. Questions about correct punctuation and spelling can be clarified through the use of a good English handbook and a standard college dictionary.

Articles submitted to professional journals for consideration for publication must follow the journals' manuscript guidelines, often displayed in the masthead or available upon request from the editorial offices. Always accompanied by a cover letter, the original article should look clean and neat, have generous margins, and be professionally typed. Occasionally, an abstract and one or two photocopies are also included. Authors must meticulously proofread their manuscripts, to catch distracting errors, before they are sent.

Editors usually inform authors within 1 or 2 months whether or not their articles have been accepted for publication. The selection process may take longer, however, if the journals are refereed or if they receive a large number of articles for consideration. Because of the need for journals to make plans well in advance to meet publishing deadlines, it is not unusual for authors to wait as long as 1 year before their articles apppear in print.

EXERCISES

1. For each of the following areas of nursing practice, list at least four journals to which you might submit an article for publication:
   - Maternal-child health
   - Public health nursing
   - Critical care nursing
   - Nursing management
   - Nursing education
   - Current trends in nursing
   - Nursing research
2. Analyze about 20 different lead paragraphs that have appeared during the past year in at least five different nursing journals. Then, give examples of four or five types of strategies that authors have used in writing leads to attract readers' attention to their articles. Do any of the strategies or techniques seem to be more effective than the others? If so, why?
3. Write a 100-word informative abstract of any nursing journal article at least 1,500 words long. Ask a colleague to read the article and your abstract and then evaluate how well the abstract summarizes the content of the article.
4. Assume that you and a colleague have completed a 2,500-word rough draft of an article entitled "Successful Strategies for Managing the Noncompliant Diabetic." Write a query letter to the editor of an appropriate journal to see whether he or she would be interested in considering the manuscript for publication.
5. Read Sandra Powell and her co-authors' article, "Writing for Publication: A Group Approach," in *Nursing Outlook,* 27 (November 1979), 729–732, to use as a starting point in discussing the advantages and disadvantages of joint authorship. Then, keeping these points in mind, write a 2,000-word paper, suitable for journal submission, with one or two members of the class or other colleagues. Work together to discuss the topic and scope of the project, the division of writing activities, and the process of journal selection. After the project is done, prepare a written critique of those items that furthered and hindered the completion of the project.

REFERENCES

1. Elida L. Mundt, "Why Don't Nurses Write?" *Nurse Educator,* 2 (March–April 1977), 6.

2. Philip C. Kolin and Janeen L. Kolin, *Professional Writing for Nurses in Education, Practice, and Research* (St. Louis: Mosby, 1980), pp. 174–177.

3. See John Herum and D. W. Cummings, *Writing: Plans, Drafts, and Revisions* (New York: Random House, 1971).

4. "Reference Sources for Nursing," *Nursing Outlook,* 28 (July 1980), 444–448.

5. Katina P. Strauch and Dorothy J. Brundage, *Guide to Library Resources in Nursing* (New York: Appleton-Century-Crofts, 1980).

6. Elizabeth Kinzer O'Farrell, "Write for the Reader, He May Need to Know What You Have to Say," *Journal of Nursing Administration,* 4 (September–October 1974), 49–53.

7. Joanne Comi McCloskey, "Publishing Opportunities for Nurses: A Comparison of 65 Journals," *Nurse Educator,* 2 (July–August 1977), 8–12.

8. Jane L. Binger, "Writing for Publication: A Survey of Nursing Journal Editors," *Journal of Nursing Administration,* 9 (January 1979), 51.

9. See William Strunk, Jr., and E. B. White, *The Elements of Style,* 3d ed. (New York: Macmillan, 1979).

10. See Jacques Barzun, *Simple and Direct: A Rhetoric for Writers* (New York: Harper & Row, 1975).

11. See Sheridan Baker, *The Practical Stylist,* 3d ed. (New York: Crowell, 1973).

12. Binger, p. 51.

13. See Mary K. Shaffer and Isobel L. Pfeiffer, "Eliminate Stereotyped Writing," *Supervisor Nurse,* 11 (April 1980), 68–70.

14. Edith P. Lewis, "What Bugs Editors," *Nursing Outlook,* 23 (August 1975), 491.

FURTHER READING

Bestor, Dorothy K. "Writing an Article for Publication: Part One." *The Nurse Practitioner,* 1 (March–April 1976), 13–17.

———. "Writing an Article for Publication: Part Two." *The Nurse Practitioner,* 1 (May–June 1976), 21–23.

Brosnan, Joan, and Andrea Kovalesky. "Perishing While Publishing: As the Authors See It." *Nursing Outlook,* 28 (November 1980), 688, 690.

Burkhalter, Pamela. "So You Want to Write." *Supervisor Nurse,* 7 (June 1976), 54–56.

Ciardi, John. "Nurses as Writers." *American Journal of Nursing,* 70 (December 1970), 2567–2570.

Evans, Nancy. "Authors and Publishers: The Mutual Selection Process." *American Journal of Nursing,* 81 (February 1981), 350–352.

Glatt, Carol R. "How Your Hospital Library Can Help You Keep Up in Nursing." *American Journal of Nursing,* 78 (April 1978), 642–644.

Hodgman, Eileen Callahan. "On Writing and Writing Workshops." *Nursing Outlook,* 28 (June 1980), 366–371.

King, Lester S. *Why Not Say It Clearly.* Boston: Little, Brown, 1978.

Lewis, Edith P. "A Peerless Publication." *Nursing Outlook,* 28 (April 1980), 225.

———. "Perishing While Publishing: As the Editor Sees It." *Nursing Outlook,* 28 (November 1980), 689–690.

———. "We're Sorry, But. . . ." *Nursing Outlook,* 21 (March 1973), 153.

Mullins, Carolyn J. *A Guide to Writing and Publishing in the Social and Behavioral Sciences.* New York: Wiley, 1977.

O'Connor, Andrea B. *Writing for Nursing Publications.* Thorofare, NJ: Slack, 1976.

Perry, Shannon E. "The Trials and Tribulations of a Would-be Author." *Supervisor Nurse,* 9 (January 1978), 13–16.

Schorr, Thelma M. "On the Subject of Writing." *American Journal of Nursing,* 77 (June 1977), 967.

Sparks, Susan M. "Letting the Computer Do the Work." *American Journal of Nursing,* 78 (April 1978), 645–647.

Stuart, Gail Wiscarz, and others. "Getting a Book Published." *Nursing Outlook,* 25 (May 1977), 316–318.

Taylor, Susan D. "How to Search the Literature." *American Journal of Nursing,* 74 (August 1974), 1457–1459.

Tobiason, Sarah Jane. "The Indexes to Nursing Literature." *Supervisor Nurse,* 9 (January 1978), 23–24.

Worthy, Elizabeth J. "Self-help for the Underpublished." *Nursing Outlook,* 19 (August 1971), 546–547.

CHAPTER VIII

Communicating About Employment In the Profession

Objectives

After studying this chapter, you will be able to

1. Prepare a self-analysis of your education, experience, activities and honors, and interests and personal qualities.
2. Make a market analysis of the available positions in a target geographical area.
3. Write a current résumé that effectively reflects your educational preparation, employment experience, and professional interests.
4. Write a letter of application for a specific or prospective opening.
5. Discuss the factors that contribute to successful employment interviews.
6. Write effective and appropriate follow-up messages: the thank-you letter, the job acceptance letter, the job refusal letter, and the letter of resignation.

Employment communications—both written and oral—are among the most important communications you send (and receive) as a professional nurse. Even as we write this chapter, unemployment and inflation are alarmingly high. But nurses are still very much in demand and able to find jobs. Why, then, should you study the communications aspect of getting a job?

We know of at least three compelling reasons. First, you may want more than just *any* job after you graduate. Second, you may want to find a *better* job later on in your career. Third, you may one day have to relocate and search for a *new* job. This chapter can help you in such situations. Too often, graduate nurses have not received guidance in this essential area of communication. Yet there is certainly a difference between (1) merely working and (2) working at the right job in a challenging atmosphere.

The six-step job-finding process we recommend to you begins with a self-analysis and market analysis, continues with your résumé and application letter, and concludes with the employment interview and follow-up messages. Knowledge of and practice in these communication steps can save you time, give you confidence, and get positive results. Effectively communicating your unique abilities and interests to the right employer at the right time can give you an edge over the competition for that "special" position.

Communicating about employment in the profession is yet another instance in which the basic principle of adaptation applies. As we proceed, you should see how the three preeminent communication facilitators of planned presentation, you-viewpoint, and appropriate language help with the six steps in the job-finding process.

SELF-ANALYSIS

A necessary first step for entering the job market the first time and each time thereafter is a self-analysis or self-appraisal in which you try to evaluate yourself from a prospective employer's point of view. What, honestly, are your employment strengths and weaknesses? What do you have that an employer should be interested in? What are your major selling points? Taking a personal inventory can help you better understand your background, more clearly come to terms with your present status, and more wisely decide what you want to do in the world of work *and* where you want to do it.

Even though no one but you might see the results of your personal inventory, doing a careful job at this stage will make the other steps in the job-finding process go more smoothly and successfully. What is your long-term goal? What are some short-term goals? These are two preliminary questions to tackle. Where in the organization do you start? Are you qualified to start? This is the time to begin thinking about making the connection between what you have done in the past (both educationally and experientially) and what you want to do next. What kind of agency would you prefer to work for? Although a hospital setting is one option, employment opportunities also exist in ambulatory care facilities, extended care facilities, public health agencies, physicians' offices, and colleges or universities. Ultimately, only you can decide.

How do you measure up in the four key areas of education, experience, activities and honors, and interests and personal qualities? For each key area, set aside a separate sheet of paper on which to write down your achievements as well as future plans or necessary improvements. Some people entering (or reentering) the job market find the plentiful checklists, tables, diagrams, and directions in Richard Nelson Bolles's somewhat lengthy book, *What Color Is Your Parachute? A Practical Manual for Job-hunters and Career-changers,* useful in completing a self-appraisal.[1] But all you really need are four large sheets of paper—one for each critical category just cited.

On the *education* sheet, you can review your knowledge base by jotting down details about schools attended, degrees earned or in progress, courses, grades, special projects or papers, and licensure, among others. Be sure to note any special courses or minors that distinguish you from others, as well as your plans for continuing your education.

On the *experience* sheet, you can summarize your work experience, skills, and abilities, especially as they are related to nursing. Your responsibilities, promotions, and percentage of school expenses earned are three items to include here.

On the *activities and honors* sheet, you can list your organizational memberships, leadership roles, academic honors, publications, convention participation, languages, and the like. By now, your uniqueness as an individual should become apparent on the worksheets before you.

On the *interests and personal qualities* sheet, you can record your attitudes toward previous courses and types of work responsibilities, small or large agencies, various geographical areas, salary, and future plans and goals. As for personal qualities, how would you rate yourself—remember, this self-analysis is for your own benefit—on such desirable characteristics as honesty, enthusiasm, problem-solving ability, cooperation, maturity, communication skill, creativity, and judgment, just to name a few? Perhaps you can use a rating scale such as A, B, C, and so on.

During this self-analysis stage of the job-finding process, therefore, you reconsider your background, capabilities, and desires with a view toward matching them with an employer's needs.

MARKET ANALYSIS

Whether you are searching for an entry-level nursing position or a more specialized, advanced position, making a market analysis is the next logical step. You need to do some careful research into the types of jobs that interest you and the kinds of employers who could use your talents.

Taking into account your preferences for agency *kind, size,* and *location,* draw up a list of prospects, that is, agencies you would like to work for. Gather specific information about each agency's history, reputation, structure, and goals. Keeping accurate and concise notes in each case will ease comparison and contrast later on.

Sources of hospital or agency information abound. Before proceeding too far in the application process—and certainly before going into an interview—you should call or write a prospective employer for its recruiting brochure. Such a brochure can answer many of your questions, provide talking points later on between you and the employer's representatives, and give you some sense of the agency's approach to nursing and nursing care delivery systems. Another information source is the agency's own annual report containing summaries of recent activities, future directions, and financial data. Talking informally with another professional who already works for an agency that interests you may help you sort out impressions and decide whether to follow through with your application. Perhaps, too, you recall (or can find) an illuminating article on a given agency in the local newspaper.

You can learn still more about the job market and obtain leads on openings through suggestions from your teachers, colleagues, and friends.

Many hospitals and agencies even send out nurse recruiters to locations (near and far) in their quest for the best-qualified personnel.

Even when you have a satisfying position, scanning the classified ads in local and out-of-town newspapers, especially in the Sunday editions, allows you to keep up with trends in the job market. And for those actively seeking positions, newspaper ads are obviously important sources of information. Spring and summer are often busy recruiting periods for both new graduates and health care institutions. Nurses relocating should, of course, subscribe to their new city's newspaper so that they can apply before actually moving. But because not all positions are advertised, you should feel free to prospect by writing or visiting an institution that particularly interests you.

Reading the employment opportunities sections of various nursing journals may also prove fruitful. Usually categorized by geographical area and/or by job title or specialty, the openings listed in *American Journal of Nursing, Nursing82, Nursing Outlook,* and *Supervisor Nurse,* for instance, can furnish some good leads for job seekers at various levels, from staff nurse through nursing service director. Moreover, nurses who are not job hunting at the moment but who may be one day can find in these nursing journals descriptions and requirements for several positions that they may want to keep on file for future reference. Nurses qualified for teaching positions should also read *The Chronicle of Higher Education,* published weekly and available by subscription or in the library.

Finally, your market analysis would not be complete without studying the annual nursing job directory published by Intermed Communications, Inc. Available at hospital and nursing school libraries and distributed free on a by-request basis to registered nurses and graduating seniors, the *Nursing80 Career Directory* offers short yet useful articles on nursing care delivery systems, specialization, relicensure, professional associations, and the job search.[2] The bulk of this 320-page resource gives detailed information on some 350 hospitals and agencies from across the country that seek qualified professional nurses. In addition to a regular RSVP service complete with several postage-paid response cards, 34 advertisers have chosen to support an "instant" RSVP service that works by means of a toll-free WATS line answering service. Major institutions are represented by generous full-page ads covering such topics as specialization, continuing education, salary and fringe benefits, working conditions, other advantages, and agency background material. We hope that the *Career Directory,* begun in 1979, flourishes during the 1980s.

Making a good market analysis allows you to adapt your eventual application to the employer's needs. This is the you-viewpoint in action— planning for sincere receiver-viewpoint communication rather than possibly selfish sender-viewpoint communication.

RÉSUMÉS

A résumé is a concise, orderly, and easy-to-read summary of your background and qualifications for professional employment. Typically one or two typed pages long, a résumé may be described as a kind of report about yourself that makes careful use of emphasis, headings, and listing. Written in outline form, a résumé succinctly yet also specifically lists and discusses (in deliberate sentence fragments) your chief qualifications. It is the key document for job seekers and job changers. You should write yours as a new graduate and then update it periodically in succeeding years. Because a special job opportunity may arise at any time, you should always have your résumé ready to show or send to a prospective employer.

After making a thoughtful self-analysis and a thorough market analysis, you are ready to prepare a résumé. Because a résumé contains data on which an application letter will be based, we strongly suggest that you write the résumé first, even though the recipient of a two-part written application will most likely read your cover letter before reviewing your résumé. Necessary for a written application package consisting of your application letter and résumé, a résumé is also useful by itself for interviews gained through a telephone call or other means. Some candidates hand the interviewer a copy of the résumé as the interview starts; other candidates send the interviewer a copy of the résumé a few days before the interview. In either case, getting your résumé into the hands of a capable interviewer can help determine what questions are asked at an interview and can help you gain some control over the eventual outcome of the job-finding process.

Since its goal is to help sell you to a prospective employer, your résumé should focus on you in an objective and honest manner, should be an essentially positive document, and should be visually attractive and eminently readable. It is one stage in convincing the employer to picture you working for him or her. Would the employer like to have the professional nurse represented by this résumé on his or her staff? The application letter, interview, and follow-up messages provide further, more explicit opportunities to develop the "what-you-can-do-for-the-employer" theme.

Review of Examples

Before we review three sample résumés, a word of caution seems in order. By all means, you should study carefully the verbal and visual features of these résumés. Indeed, you can use them as aids in getting started on a successful résumé of your own. But you should avoid simply copying anyone else's résumé, for that practice would probably not do justice to your

```
RESUME              JANICE P. FULTON


PERSONAL            Home Address:  1189 Market Avenue
                                   Kent, Ohio  44126
                    Telephone:     (216) 853-2119

REGISTRATION        Will take Ohio State Boards in June 1981

EDUCATION           B.S.N., Kent State University, June 1981; won Kent Nursing
                    Scholarship, 1980-81; made Dean's List, 7 quarters;
                    completed clinical nursing experience at Kent General
                    Hospital and Akron City Hospital

EMPLOYMENT          Research Assistant, Kent State University, November 1980-
                    June 1981; responsible for searching card catalog and
                    nursing periodicals on various topics assigned by several
                    nursing professors and for writing abstracts of promising
                    sources
                    Nursing Assistant, Kent General Hospital, Psychiatric Unit,
                    October 1977-October 1980

SPECIAL FIELDS      Psychiatric Nursing; Geriatric Nursing
OF INTEREST

PROFESSIONAL        National Student Nurses Association
ORGANIZATIONS

CIVIC               Telephone Volunteer, Kent County Rape Crisis Center, 1980-81
ORGANIZATIONS

WORKSHOPS           "Beginning Management Skills for Nurses," Cleveland State
ATTENDED            University, May 1-2, 1981
                    "Psychiatric Nursing:  The State of the Art," University of
                    Akron, November 29, 1980
                    "New Directions in Geriatric Nursing," Kent General Hospital,
                    March 15, 1980

PUBLICATIONS        "The Psychiatric Nurse and the Law," a problem forthcoming in
                    the Advice, p.r.n. section of Nursing81

REFERENCES          Dorothy T. Green, R.N., M.S.N.    Joseph A. Hill, R.N.
                    Assistant Professor of Nursing    Head Nurse, Psychiatric Unit
                    Kent State University             Kent General Hospital
                    Kent, Ohio  44120                 Kent, Ohio  44128

                    Marie H. Johns, R.N., B.S.N.      Nancy C. Zesmer, R.N., Ph.D.
                    Instructor in Nursing             Associate Professor of Nursing
                    Kent State University             Kent State University
                    Kent, Ohio  44120                 Kent, Ohio  44120
```

Exhibit 8.1. A new graduate's résumé.

uniqueness as a person and as a professional. Instead, we suggest that after examining the samples and then assimilating the guidelines that follow, you strike out on your own to discover the best wording, plan, and format to do justice to *your* background and qualifications. There are many features that all résumés have in common, but there is no reason why all résumés must read or look exactly alike.

Exhibit 8.1 is a general-purpose one-page résumé of a new graduate. It effectively employs attractive side headings, capitalization, and white space. Ms. Fulton first identifies herself and supplies essential personal data; then she concisely explains her registration status. Her educational background receives emphasis here, as it should for most recent graduates. Next comes relevant work experience, listed in reverse chronological order and interpreted where necessary and desirable. Ms. Fulton lists two special fields of interest, namely, psychiatric nursing and geriatric nursing. Her résumé could be used to apply to several health care agencies (near and far) where an entry-level position might exist in one or the other of these clinical areas she wishes to pursue. A summary of her organizational memberships and workshops attended (with specific titles, place, and date for each) rounds out the presentation. She has one short piece accepted for publication. And four professionally relevant references are listed at the end, three from university professors who know her well and one from her former head nurse. Of course, Ms. Fulton has secured her referees' permission *before* including them on her résumé. She gives a generally good account of herself at this stage in her professional development. Although résumés are not dated (as are letters), this document clearly was prepared during June 1981. It is ready for professional duplication; offset printing of this camera-ready résumé would, for a nominal cost, allow for multiple submissions without repetitive retyping.

The second résumé, as shown in Exhibit 8.2, is a personalized one-page résumé of an experienced practitioner. Because Mr. Cole uses an individually tailored headline opening to match a job he knows has just opened up, this particular résumé page cannot be duplicated and sent to several employers. This applicant's objective and potential employer are clear from the start. He provides his address and telephone number, then quickly launches into professional experience, his central selling point. Educational experience follows; his registration, nearly completed B.S.N., and A.A.S. reveal his progress in nursing education to date. Papers delivered give an even clearer picture of this candidate's accomplishments and areas of expertise. Seminars and workshops, as well as appropriate professional memberships, conclude the presentation. References "will be furnished upon request," for Mr. Cole is applying to Austin Memorial Hospital confidentially. Should his candidacy there flourish, he will then want to provide references for the head nurse position after first speaking with selected colleagues at Green County Hospital, where he

```
            FRANK X. COLE'S QUALIFICATIONS FOR HEAD NURSE,

            ORTHOPEDICS, AT AUSTIN MEMORIAL HOSPITAL


                        597 Cynthia Street
                        Apartment #7
                        Austin, Texas  78748
                        Telephone 443-6710


                        Professional Experience

Senior Primary Nurse, Green County Hospital, Austin, Neuro-orthopedics Unit,
    1979-present
Staff Nurse, Green County Hospital, Rehabilitation Unit, 1978-79
Staff Nurse, Green County Hospital, Intensive Care Unit, 1977-78
Operating Room Technician, Dallas General Hospital, 1975-77
Surgical Technician, U.S. Munson Army Hospital, Ft. Leavenworth, Kansas,
    1974-75

                        Educational Experience

Registration:  Q 327891 Texas
B.S.N., University of Texas, Austin, expected December 1981
A.A.S., Dallas Community College, June 1977

                        Papers Delivered

"Postoperative Nursing Care of the Patient with Dupuytren's Contracture,"
    Texas Orthopedic Nurses Association, Green County Chapter, November 13, 1980
"The Rehabilitation Nurse's Role in Bowel and Bladder Training," part of an
    eight-hour Workshop on the Hazards of Immobility, Green County Hospital,
    February 21, 1979

                        Workshops and Seminars

"Coping with the Alcoholic's Behavior," Austin Memorial Hospital, March 28, 1981
"Advanced Concepts in Nursing Management," Baylor University, Waco, May 5-9, 1980
"Sexuality and Aging:  Implications for Long-Term Care," St. Anthony's
    Hospital, Ft. Worth, July 7, 1978
"Adult Physical Assessment," University of Texas, Austin, June-August 1977

                        Professional Memberships

American Nurses Association
Texas Orthopedic Nurses Association
Association of Rehabilitation Nurses

                        References

Will be furnished upon request
```

Exhibit 8.2. An experienced practitioner's résumé.

```
RESUME          ELAINE M. KOZIER


PERSONAL        Home Address:    17 Millersville Drive
                                 Seattle, Washington  98106
                Telephone:       (206) 252-0004

REGISTRATION    L 576112 Washington; T 301079 Illinois

EDUCATION       M.S.N., University of Washington, June 1979; specialized in
                  maternal-child health nursing
                B.S.N., University of Illinois, Chicago Circle, June 1975;
                  graduated magna cum laude
                Diploma, Rockford Memorial Hospital School of Nursing,
                  June 1970

AWARDS AND      Nursing Faculty Award for Outstanding Graduate Research,
HONORS            University of Washington, June 1979
                Sigma Theta Tau, University of Illinois, elected December 1974
                Dean's List, University of Illinois, 6 semesters

EMPLOYMENT      Head Nurse, Swedish Hospital Medical Center, Seattle,
                  Family-Centered Care Unit, 1979-present
                Adjunct Instructor in Nursing, University of Washington,
                  January 1980-present
                Assistant Head Nurse, Swedish Hospital Medical Center,
                  Special Care Nursery, 1975-78
                Staff Nurse, Rush-Presbyterian-St. Luke's Medical Center,
                  Chicago, Newborn Nursery, 1973-75
                Team Leader, Rockford Memorial Hospital, Pediatrics Unit,
                  1972-73
                Staff Nurse, Rockford Memorial Hospital, Medical Unit,
                  1970-72

ORGANIZATIONAL  National League for Nursing
MEMBERSHIPS     American Nurses Association
                Washington State Nurses Association
                Association for the Care of Children in Hospitals
                Task Force on Maternal-Child Health, Advisory Committee,
                  Washington State Nurses Association

RECENT          "Beyond Childbirth--Social Change:  Its Impact on Infants
WORKSHOPS         and Their Care-Givers," Santa Barbara, California,
ATTENDED          April 4-6, 1981
                "Care of the Critically Ill Child," University of Washington,
                  January-February 1981
                "Research for Clinical Nursing:  Its Strategies and Findings,"
                  University of Idaho, November 20, 1980
```

Exhibit 8.3. Résumé for a teaching position.

```
RESUME              ELAINE M. KOZIER                                    PAGE 2


RESEARCH            "The Physiological Effects of Touch on Low-Birth-Weight
                       Neonates Receiving Continuous Transcutaneous Oxygen
                       Therapy," University of Washington, M.S.N. Thesis,
                       June 1979

PUBLICATIONS        "Monitoring Transcutaneous Oxygen Tension in Hypoxic
                       Neonates," forthcoming in Nursing Research

REFERENCES          Gretchen V. Brown, R.N., M.N.A.
                    Director of Nursing
                    Swedish Hospital Medical Center
                    Seattle, Washington  98133

                    Lilian D. Crawford, R.N., Ph.D.
                    Professor of Nursing
                    University of Washington
                    Seattle, Washington  98142

                    Paul O. Duncan, R.N., M.S.N.
                    Associate Professor of Nursing
                    University of Washington
                    Seattle, Washington  98142

                    Regina Holmes Gent, R.N., M.S.N.
                    Associate Professor of Nursing
                    University of Illinois, Chicago Circle
                    Chicago, Illinois  60678
```

Exhibit 8.3.   (Continued)

now works, and with other potential referees. This résumé makes fine use of centered, underlined headings and generous white space. It adapts well to the job opening in its form and specific content.

The third résumé, as shown in Exhibit 8.3, is a two-page résumé for a teaching position. Ms. Kozier is registered in Washington and Illinois. Her education, especially her M.S.N., is a key qualification that receives deserved emphasis here. Her awards and honors reveal academic excellence and special recognition for nursing research. Her employment history is crisply presented, and her two most recent positions of head nurse and adjunct instructor in nursing especially support her candidacy for a faculty position. Her memberships are appropriate, and two directly support her specialty, maternal-child health nursing. Only workshops attended recently are listed. There will be time in the interview for Ms. Kozier to say more about herself than just two typed pages can contain. But her research and publications together make for a strong finale for the faculty position she seeks, for these qualifications are especially important to her future success as a faculty member. References are impressive—two professors from the University of Washington, one professor from the University of Illinois, and her current director of nursing, who knows she is seeking a full-time faculty position. Sometimes you will see the terms *curriculum vitae* or *vita* used for résumés, such as Ms. Kozier's, that are geared toward applying for academic positions.

Guidelines for Writing Résumés

Whether you are a recent graduate, an experienced practitioner, or a candidate for a teaching position, a carefully prepared résumé can introduce you to several possible employers. Because your résumé changes as you develop professionally, it should be revised and updated periodically. A new degree, a promotion, a publication—these are just some of the accomplishments you will want your résumé to reflect as they occur. But there is no single format for a résumé. Looking at the samples just analyzed and applying the 10 guidelines discussed next should enable you to develop the résumé that best *fits you* and *sells you* to best advantage.

Guideline 1
Begin your résumé with the label *résumé* and your name both in capital letters at the top of the page. Sometimes a more specifically informative headline opening may be appropriate for certain application situations. "QUALIFICATIONS OF CHRIS W. BONNER AS HOME HEALTH NURSE" and "DAWN A. TOLSON'S QUALIFICATIONS FOR STAFF NURSE AT MADISON CITIZENS HOSPITAL" are two examples. General-purpose résumés may be professionally duplicated and sent to several agencies, whereas personalized résumés that refer to a prospective employer by name in the headline can be used for that employer only and must be retyped each time you send one.

Guideline 2
After your name, give essential personal data such as address and telephone number. Modern résumés rarely include a photograph or such items as sex, age, race, national origin, religion, health, or marital status. You may, of course, choose to volunteer such information; but employers cannot use it to deny you a job in light of such legislation as the 1964 Civil Rights Act, the 1967 Age Discrimination Act, and the 1972 Equal Employment Opportunity Act. We think that providing more than the essentials of name, address, and telephone number is, quite frankly, not worth the space it would take on a résumé, especially when so many other important topics require coverage.

Guideline 3
Follow personal data with sections on education, registration, employment, special fields of interest or experience, organizational member-

ships, and references. When you have accomplishments or activities in other categories such as awards and honors, papers delivered, workshops attended, research, and publications, be sure to incorporate them into your résumé under appropriate headings.

Guideline 4

Emphasize early your central selling point of education or experience. New graduates and potential faculty members usually lead with education followed by experience. Experienced practitioners applying for non-academic jobs usually lead with work experience followed by education. The rationale here is to emphasize your strongest qualification for a certain area of work by positioning it close to the beginning of the résumé, where the reader will readily spot it.

Guideline 5

List in separate sections and in reverse chronological order (from most recent to least recent) your educational experience, work experience, papers delivered, workshops attended, and so on. This procedure allows busy readers to find out easily and quickly what they most want to know about you.

Guideline 6

Type your résumé on an electric typewriter, preferably one equipped with a black carbon ribbon. For a professional appearance, choose quality 8½" × 11", white, 20-lb stationery. Select only a quality duplicating process, such as offset printing, for a general-purpose résumé to be sent to more than one employer. Identify and number pages after the first. Staple a two-page résumé once in the upper left corner.

Guideline 7

Because a résumé is a tabulation in outline form, avoid lengthy paragraphs and complete sentences. Use phrases or deliberate sentence fragments to get more information on the page. Personal pronouns, particularly *I* and *you*, should not appear on a résumé because of the need for conciseness and objectivity. Instead, focus on facts and qualifications, and keep opinions and repetition out of the résumé.

Guideline 8

Balance material across the page in tabulated form. Capitalizing side headings or underlining centered headings makes a résumé readable and attractive. Use hanging indention when you have to carry over an item beyond one line within a category such as education, employment, workshops, and the like. Also, be consistent in the layout, as are the individual authors of the three sample résumés discussed previously.

Guideline 9
Observe parallel construction in outlining and listing. Thus, headings should be parallel and succinct. And the items within each category should be parallel so that, for instance, under "Employment" each item contains title of position, name of employer, unit, and dates. Moreover, parallel "action" verbs should be used within sections to indicate accomplishments and responsibilities. Some examples are

- Administered
- Coordinated
- Developed
- Evaluated
- Finished
- Increased
- Led
- Planned
- Scheduled
- Trained
- Won
- Wrote

Guideline 10
Check for accuracy in facts, mechanics, and spelling. Proofread carefully for a letter-perfect résumé worthy of a nurse professional. Whether you think it fair or not, résumé readers make a judgment about you on the basis of what they see on the page. Many interviewers tell us that carelessness on the résumé makes them wonder whether a prospective employee will be equally careless on the job. Don't give employers anything with which to "screen you out"!

APPLICATION LETTERS

When you have occasion to apply for a position by mail, you send an original application letter—always individually typed, specifically adapted to the agency that interests you, and customarily one page long—as well as a copy of your up-to-date résumé.

The application letter, the fourth stage in the six-step job-finding process, should be viewed as an informative *sales letter* with you, in a sense, as the "product." This important persuasive letter reveals much about you as it seeks to (1) gain, at the outset, the reader's attentive interest in your candidacy, (2) develop the reader's desire to hear even more about your good qualifications in light of the convincing evidence presented in your letter's body, and (3) lead the reader, by means of your action ending, to call you soon for an interview. Developed around a central selling point of education, experience, or a special combination of features likely to induce the reader to pursue your candidacy, the application letter, therefore, employs the three planned steps of successful selling—attentive interest, desire or conviction, and action ending.

Furthermore, an application letter is solicited when an agency invites candidates to apply for an announced opening. In this case, your letter-résumé package is expected (along with perhaps many others). An application letter is unsolicited when you do not know an opening exists yet you decide to prospect by communicating with an agency that interests you. The three different application letters that follow will clarify the solicited-unsolicited distinction, exemplify the three selling steps in action, and illustrate three nurses' approaches to this highly creative form of written communication about employment in the profession.

Review of Examples

Exhibit 8.4 is the cover letter that accompanies Janice P. Fulton's résumé (see Exhibit 8.1). Her fairly complete prospecting application possesses a sincere you-viewpoint and appropriate language, for it talks work and doing in reader-benefit terms. The letter is well planned, also. Attentive interest is achieved in the opening paragraph when the writer asks a pertinent question, applies for the hoped-for position, and summarizes her three qualifications. Desire or conviction is engendered in the three body paragraphs, one each on education, experience, and job-related interests. Here Ms. Fulton amplifies, through reader-oriented paragraphs and complete sentences, selected portions of her résumé; she focuses on her background *and* what she can do with it on the job at Mount Carmel. The last paragraph mentions the résumé—and what the reader will get from it—and confidently asks for an interview at the reader's convenience. This letter's format is traditional, conservative, and attractive. Should the writer receive a positive reply, she would appear to be ready for a meeting with Ms. Droll in Columbus. Certainly, this applicant has done her homework on Mount Carmel, and she directs the application to the one person with the power to hire her.

The second application letter, as shown in Exhibit 8.5, complements Frank X. Cole's résumé (see Exhibit 8.2). This letter is solicited, for Austin Memorial advertised in the Sunday *Times Herald*. In this case, however, Mr. Cole wisely decided first to call Mrs. Turner about the head nurse opening. Then he followed their conversation with his formal appli-

```
                                            1189 Market Avenue
                                            Kent, Ohio  44126
                                            June 4, 1981

Ms. Karen Droll, R.N.
Nurse Recruiter
Mount Carmel Medical Center
793 West State Street
Columbus, Ohio  43222

Dear Ms. Droll:

Later this summer will your psychiatric unit need a beginning staff nurse
who can establish solid lines of communication with each client in a
sensitive and professional manner?  If so, please consider me for the
position.  My qualifications include a sound nursing background, relevant
experience, and a special interest in psychiatric nursing.

To prepare myself for a career in professional nursing, I have completed
work on my B.S.N. at Kent State University, graduating on June 2 with a
grade point average of 3.6 (on a 4-point scale).  Two senior-level
nursing courses to which I devoted much time and effort--Psychiatric/
Mental Health Nursing and Nursing of Adults with Complex Health Problems--
will help me in working with clients on your psychiatric unit.  I am
scheduled to take Ohio State Boards on June 29 and can begin work soon
after that date.

Three years as a nursing assistant on Kent General Hospital's psychiatric
unit and almost eight months as a research assistant at Kent State working
mostly on topics in psychiatric and geriatric nursing have given me
valuable insight into current nursing practice and theory.  One year's
telephone volunteer work at the Kent County Rape Crisis Center strengthened
my interpersonal communication skills, skills which you know are so
important to effective psychiatric nursing.

At an institution like Mount Carmel that emphasizes psychiatric care and
is licensed by the Department of Mental Health and Mental Retardation, I
believe that I could successfully develop in this clinical area.  A short
article forthcoming for Nursing81 and a November 1980 workshop I attended
demonstrate, in part, my interest in and commitment to psychiatric nursing.

After you have had an opportunity to review my qualifications and contact
the references listed on the enclosed resume, won't you write or call me,
naming a time when we can talk further about how I could help on your
psychiatric unit?

                                            Sincerely,


Enclosure:  Resume                          Janice P. Fulton
```

Exhibit 8.4. A new graduate's application letter.

597 Cynthia Street
Apartment #7
Austin, Texas   78748
April 30, 1981

Mrs. Kate D. Turner, R.N.
Director of Nursing
Austin Memorial Hospital
2784 Spicetree Boulevard
Austin, Texas   78752

Dear Mrs. Turner:

Because of our productive conversation this morning about your ad in
the Sunday Times Herald, I remain very interested in Austin Memorial's
opening for a head nurse of orthopedics. As I promised, here is my
current resume for your review before our meeting next week.

Briefly, I feel that my experience--both professional and educational--
qualifies me for the head nurse position. For the past two years I have
served as senior primary nurse on Green County Hospital's neuro-
orthopedics unit, and by December I will have completed all requirements
for the B.S.N. from the University of Texas. Since becoming a registered
nurse in 1977, I have been active both in attending workshops and in
delivering papers. Now, becoming a member of the progressive nursing
management team at Austin Memorial seems like the logical next step in
my career.

In short, I look forward, Mrs. Turner, to our 4 p.m. meeting next
Wednesday when we can discuss further your requirements and my
qualifications for the head nurse position.

                                        Sincerely,

Enclosure: Resume   Frank X. Cole, R.N.

Exhibit 8.5. An experienced practitioner's transmittal.

cation and résumé. In fact, his letter is a transmittal, since he uses it to
convey a bit more information about himself (beyond the telephone conversation) and to get the résumé into Mrs. Turner's hands. Although
shorter than some other application letters you might see, it still contains
the three selling steps. The first paragraph gains attentive interest
through its reference to their conversation and to the newspaper ad. It
whets the reader's appetite to learn more from the résumé. Basic conviction is generated by the overview of qualifications in the second paragraph. Mr. Cole makes a generally good case for his head nurse candidacy. The action ending with its personalized language ("I look forward,
Mrs. Turner, to . . .") recalls the specifics of next week's meeting and adds
a last punch line on reader benefit. Mr. Cole is nicely positioned for his
interview with Mrs. Turner.

17 Millersville Drive
Seattle, Washington 98106
May 22, 1981

Professor C. V. Warren
Dean, College of Nursing
Northern Illinois University
DeKalb, Illinois 60118

Dear Professor Warren:

Faculty position for M.S.N. with experience . . . specialty area in maternal-child health nursing . . . appropriate research and publication plans. . . .

These key words from your May 21 advertisement in The Chronicle of Higher Education describe the person you want, and I believe I am that person.

With an M.S.N. earned from the University of Washington, intensive graduate work in maternal-child health nursing, and recent experience both as a head nurse of a family-centered care unit and as an adjunct instructor in nursing, I am confident that I could contribute significantly to your revised and expanding program. Because I have family ties in the northern Illinois area, I would feel "at home" in DeKalb. My interest in teaching has developed in the past several years as I completed my M.S.N. work and rose from staff nurse to head nurse--a position itself that carries a good deal of teaching responsibility. My part-time teaching for the University of Washington has been so rewarding that I now seek to make this career transition.

As you will see from the attached resume, my thesis on low-birth-weight neonates won the 1979 Nursing Faculty Award for Outstanding Graduate Research. My article, "Monitoring Transcutaneous Oxygen Tension in Hypoxic Neonates," has been accepted by Nursing Research. Other related research projects are under way.

Because I will be visiting in Rockford from May 30 to June 6, I would appreciate the opportunity to see you during that time to discuss further my desire to serve as your new faculty member in maternal-child health nursing. You can reach me in the evening by calling (216) 252-0004.

Sincerely,

Enclosure: Resume   Elaine M. Kozier, R.N., M.S.N.

Exhibit 8.6. Application letter for a teaching position.

The third letter, as shown in Exhibit 8.6, exemplifies the more complete type of application, and it accompanies Elaine M. Kozier's two-page résumé (see Exhibit 8.3). This solicited application for a teaching position uses a somewhat aggressive, yet rather effective, combination summary-of-qualifications and name-of-source opening based on Professor Warren's own ad in *The Chronicle of Higher Education*. After the initial two paragraphs arouse attention and interest, Ms. Kozier supplies two body paragraphs to convince the reader that her claim to be "the person" for the job has considerable merit. She adapts well to the academic position, the university, and the geographical area. Her final paragraph respectfully asks for action, explains who does what next, and stresses a can-do attitude.

Guidelines for Writing Application Letters

If you now carefully reconsider those three application letters (and their accompanying résumés) from nurses with different backgrounds, qualifications, and goals, and if you also apply these six guidelines for writing application letters, you should be better prepared to respond to the more likely employment communication situations you might encounter in the future. Once again, however, we caution against merely copying anyone else's application. Put your ideas in your own words as you follow these guidelines for writing.

Guideline 1
Because appearance and accuracy count in your letter just as they do in your résumé, go back and review the sixth and tenth guidelines for writing résumés. Those suggestions apply equally well to application letters, except for the advice on duplicating a general-purpose résumé. Your letter must *never* be duplicated; each one you send should be individually typed and adapted to a specific agency or employer. You can probably fit on one typed page, with at least 1¼" margins on all sides, all you need to highlight about your qualifications. The letter, written in receiver-oriented paragraphs and sentences, develops selected points outlined on the résumé. All three sample letters use the conservative, traditional layout of a standard business letter as a vehicle for individual, unique content.[3]

Guideline 2
Begin the letter with your return address and the date at the right. Double-space (skip two lines). Then at the left margin, supply the name and title of the addressee, the agency, and its address. Double-space again. Then make the salutation—for example, "Dear Ms. Droll." Writing directly to the one person with the power to hire you is better than writing to "Dear Sir or Madam" or "Dear Nurse Recruiter." In an article about employment communications, Mary C. Parker aptly suggests that besides researching various placement directories and, when available, classified ads, you can even "place a phone call to the organization's switchboard to find out the name"[4] of the person to contact. Double-space after the salutation and you are ready for the message itself.

The paragraphs in the letter are blocked at the left margin, with a double space separating them. Close the letter with *Sincerely,* lined up at the right with your return address at the top. Skip four lines; type your name; then sign in ink in the signature block (between the close and your typed name). At the left, opposite your typed name, the enclosure notation should appear to help you remember to enclose your résumé and to help your reader remember to look at it.

Guideline 3

Whether the letter is solicited or unsolicited, a complete application or a somewhat shorter transmittal, employ the three planned steps of successful selling—attentive interest, desire or conviction, and action ending. Your opening paragraph can pose a reader-benefit question or summarize your main qualifications or refer by name to an ad you read or a person who told you about the job, as you simultaneously apply for the specific position or field of interest. Devoting from one to three paragraphs to (1) discussing your education, experience, and special interests in terms of doing something for the reader or agency and to (2) telling why you want to work for that agency helps bring about desire on the reader's part to hear more. After you convince the reader of the merits of your candidacy, a subtly subordinated reference to your résumé (stressing especially what the reader can get from it, not the fact that it is enclosed) and a confident request for a meeting to discuss further what you can contribute as an employee conclude the persuasive effort.

Guideline 4

Weave your research *gracefully* into the letter. In addition to addressing the application to the right person in the organization, you can add personalized language once or twice toward the end by mentioning the reader's name ("In short, Ms. Ely, I feel that . . ."). You can also talk agency trends and operations ("At an institution like Mercy Hospital that emphasizes pediatric nursing . . ." or "I could contribute . . . to your revised and growing program").

Guideline 5

In order to maintain naturalness in the letter, feel free to use the personal pronouns *I* and *you* as necessary and appropriate—but not to excess. Using *I* too many times can sound selfish; using *you* too many times can sound too familiar. Moderation is best here.

Guideline 6

End the letter with a clear statement of who does what next and with a final punch line on reader benefit. You don't want to be presumptuous ("What time can I see you next Thursday?"), but neither do you want to be unsure of yourself or overly general ("If you think I could qualify, can we meet sometime?"). Usually, you ask the employer to call or write so that a mutually convenient meeting can be set up to discuss, face to face, how you can fulfill the organization's specific professional needs.

EMPLOYMENT INTERVIEWS

A special occasion for sharing information and attitudes is one good way of defining the term *interview*. Ideally, an interview should be a two-way communication situation between the interviewer (who asks questions and listens carefully) and the interviewee (who also asks questions and listens carefully). As an applicant for a nursing position, you not only *answer questions* about your background, qualifications, and goals but also *ask questions* about the specific position, about how your goals fit in with the agency's future, about advancement, and about continuing education.

Since you have already made a self-analysis and a market analysis as well as written a résumé and (probably) an application letter (or, depending on the circumstances, a transmittal), you are actually better prepared for a face-to-face meeting with the employer than you may at first realize. You certainly have the advantage over those applicants who have not followed any sort of systematic job-finding plan, such as the one discussed in this chapter.

New graduates will usually want to interview with several agencies in order to discover the right job to start with and the best place to work. In a positive sense, it pays to be "a comparison job hunter,"[5] according to a recent Career Advice column in *Nursing80*. The employment interview can help you (and the employer) decide whether a good match seems likely.

In many organizations, a nurse recruiter conducts an initial screening interview that may or may not take place at the agency itself. After such a preliminary interview, you may then be asked to a second, perhaps longer, interview with your prospective head nurse or director of nursing. A tour of the facilities, with an opportunity to meet various people and see firsthand the kind of care given, may also be incorporated into the interviewing process.

Of course, different agencies follow different procedures. Some may interview you once for an hour, then make a decision on the job right away. Others may require two separate interviews yet still need to have some more time before calling you with a decision. And applicants for teaching positions can expect an initial credentials review before meeting with the dean, the faculty, or perhaps even the students. Whatever interview procedures you encounter, however, ought to be characterized by fairness to both sides of this important two-way communication situation.

Whether interviewing is new to you or an experience you have encountered several times, you can profit from reviewing the suggestions on what to do before, during, and after an interview.

The Preinterview Phase

First, from notes you made during the market analysis, you can review the information you have already gathered about the agency. But can you learn even more about this organization before your interview? Also, who is the interviewer—his or her name, background, special interests?

Next, you should think about the kinds of questions you might be asked and how you would respond to them. Here is a list of 15 questions frequently asked during interviews:

1. Why do you want to work for us?
2. Why have you chosen this particular field of nursing?
3. Tell me about yourself.
4. What have you learned from your previous jobs?
5. How was your education financed?
6. What is your idea of successful nursing?
7. Why do you want to leave your present job?
8. What is your greatest strength?
9. Name some of your short-term goals.
10. How does your experience—educational and work—prepare you for a position such as this one?
11. Did you enjoy your schooling?
12. Why did you choose nursing as your profession?
13. What is important to you in a job?
14. What do you expect to be doing in nursing 5 years from now?
15. What are your plans for continued study?

Third, you should write down some of *your own* questions about the agency and the position, for you will have a chance during the interview to do more than answer questions. You can ask about policies and procedures for orientation, promotion, and transfers. Questions on staffing patterns and client care assignments are also appropriate. Referring to your own short list of questions at the interview will show organization and preparation.

Finally, you can ask for and fill out in advance any job application form the agency has. But because no form can replace your own résumé—designed to *sell you*—you would do well to send a letter-résumé package to the employer, if you have not already done so.

Double checking the time and place of the meeting and getting a good night's sleep before the interview are two confidence-building steps that conclude the preinterview phase.

The Interview Phase

The expression "first impressions count" may sound a bit clichéd, yet personnel experts testify to its continued validity. How you look and how you act from the outset are part of the communication context of the interview.

Punctuality, composure, businesslike appearance, courtesy, and good eye contact always work in your favor. Essentially, you try to eliminate or minimize noise sources or distractions during the interview. Being on time is easy if you plan ahead and allow time for traffic and the like. Relaxing and enjoying this professional meeting is something that may come naturally or may come only after several interviews. Dressing in a neat, businesslike manner remains solid advice for professionals seeking employment. Good manners are a must, as you try to persuade the interviewer that you would be an asset to the agency. Maintaining good eye contact without staring also favorably impresses interviewers. And because body language communicates, you should remember that posture, facial expressions, gestures, and even handshakes can reveal much about you. Fidgeting, smoking, and chewing gum are possible communication barriers best avoided. Listening well, responding clearly and completely, and showing interest in the business at hand are qualities to develop.

We agree with the advice on positive aspect and listener benefit that appears in the *Nursing79 Career Directory*. On the one hand, you should stress positive features and subordinate the negative where you legitimately can. For example, "Don't criticize former employers or co-workers. Don't give any long, drawn-out explanations or hard-luck stories."[6] On the other hand, you should emphasize something for the listener before you bring up something for yourself. The hint contained in the statement that "Interviewers are impressed with applicants who ask first about patient care, clinical areas, and staffing policies. Those who ask first about salary, benefits, and promotions have a strike against them"[7] is well worth taking. Even though you have a justifiable interest in the second three items listed, the employer understandably finds the first three—and your reactions to them—more important to the hiring process. You would do well to adapt to the interviewer's viewpoint here, even as you maintain a degree of balanced self-interest at the same time.

When the interview ends, you will want to agree on who does what next. Will a decision come soon? How long will you have to accept if an offer is forthcoming? Sometimes, of course, you may be offered the job on the spot and decide to accept. Usually, a written confirmation of your beginning date, assignment, schedule, and salary follows an oral offer.

The Postinterview Phase

After you leave an interview, you should take a few minutes to record your impressions. How well do you think things went? What did you do well? What not so well? This kind of self-evaluation can aid you in future interviews. Writing down the names of those you met and any new information gained about the agency or the position is effort well spent. The interviewer has now gained information about you on which to base a decision; you in turn need to weigh what you have learned before deciding whether you really want to pursue your candidacy after the interview.

The postinterview phase, therefore, can lead you into several follow-up messages.

FOLLOW-UP MESSAGES

The sixth and last stage to look at in the job-finding process consists of follow-up messages. Our review of the four main types of follow-up messages reveals the way several applicants handled well various written messages at this stage. But before considering the thank-you letter, the job acceptance letter, the job refusal letter, and the letter of resignation, we need to understand two special cases.

On the one hand, if you have prospected by mail with an application letter and résumé but have not received a reply within about 3 weeks, you can send a short follow-up letter reselling yourself and signalling your continued interest in the agency. This message follows up on your first mailing and tries to gain a response—hopefully a favorable one— from an agency that really interests you. This new letter of inquiry does not repeat what was in the first, nor do you include another résumé. Instead, the second letter contains a reference to the position sought, the date you sent the original letter-résumé package, any new material you can cite about your qualifications, your telephone number, and another offer to meet with the employer at a convenient time. Often, this resale follow-up brings promising results, as you tactfully communicate your continued interest in working for the employer.

A second special situation calls for a thank-you note even when the interview seems unfavorable and/or when you are no longer interested in working for that agency. This message can maintain good will and foster good human relations if you include sincere gratitude for the time the employer spent in meeting with you, specific appreciation for the frank discussion held on the duties of the position, a word or two on your plans to apply to an agency perhaps more suited to your special talents or interests, and a closing wish that the employer find the right person to fill the job you applied for. Sending a thank-you letter after *every* interview, whether things went well or not, is the courteous and professional thing to do. After all, the interviewer has devoted a portion of his or her time to meet with you.

The Thank-You Letter

When the interview goes fairly well, a decision is pending, and you still want to work for an especially appealing agency, you send a sincere, direct, and prompt thank-you letter. Your goal is to thank the interviewer for speaking with you and to recap your qualifications, as in the following message:

> Thank you very much for taking the time to meet with me yesterday. Our discussion of Mercy Hospital's recently established psychiatric unit was both informative and interesting, and I remain eager to make a contribution to it as a staff nurse.
>
> As you will recall, I recently completed work on my B.S.N. at the University of Kansas, took state boards on July 15, and spent the last 2 years as a full-time nursing assistant on Kansas City General Hospital's psychiatric unit.
>
> Please call me if I can provide further information about my education and experience. In the meantime, I know you will consider me carefully—and, I hope, favorably—for the position we discussed.

Such a letter helps distinguish you from the competition, for surprisingly few applicants take the time to send a thank-you letter. But writing a good one is not hard, and the message can be quite impressive.

The Job Acceptance Letter

Your letter accepting a job offer should be an immediate message that begins with the good news and that seals the contract. The following letter is a good example:

> Yes, I do want to work as the assistant head nurse on Mississippi Baptist Medical Center's newborn intensive care unit, and I'm pleased to accept your offer.
>
> The conditions specified in your letter of February 5, including responsibilities, schedule, and salary, are all agreeable to me. I've enclosed the completed medical and insurance forms you sent.
>
> Because I know I'll be able to justify your confidence in me, I look forward to reporting for work on Monday, March 1.

A job acceptance letter, then, is direct, courteous, enthusiastic, and specific about terms and dates. It also lets you restate your interest in serving the employer well.

The Job Refusal Letter

Declining a job offer is somewhat harder than accepting one. An indirect or delayed message strategy that (1) opens with some favorable comment about the employer or the work, (2) moves into a careful explanation or reasoning section about the decision to come, (3) states subordinately and positively this decision, and (4) adds a pleasant, friendly closing is preferable in this potentially good will–killing situation:

> It was a pleasure to meet with you and talk over the details of the teaching position you are seeking to fill. In addition, I was gratified to receive your offer last week.
>
> As you know from our conversation, I am still primarily interested in working in a B.S.N. degree program with students who are already registered nurses with diploma or associate-degree backgrounds. Even though I am now completing my doctorate, I feel a special affinity with today's nongeneric graduates, since I entered nursing through an associate-degree program.
>
> After seriously considering your fine offer and the fact that your university focuses almost exclusively on generic students' needs, I have finally decided to accept a position at Rootstown State University, where baccalaureate nursing for registered nurses only is offered.
>
> Thank you again, Dean Olds, for your interest in me.

The preceding letter is tactful and, above all, reader-oriented, for although Dean Olds has other qualified candidates to turn to, she still spent considerable time and effort on this applicant. But when people are shown the legitimate reasons behind a refusal, they will usually accept it.

The Letter of Resignation

Like the job refusal letter, the letter of resignation is a bad-news message that usually calls for the delayed or indirect structure (reasons *before* decision). In this case, however, you should first discuss your resignation with your superior. Then you follow up with a good will–retaining letter, such as the following one from an emergency room nurse to the head nurse:

> My three years as an emergency room nurse at Lawnwood Medical Center have been stimulating and rewarding.
>
> I will always be grateful to you and the other professionals at Lawnwood who have helped me to do the job and to prepare for an even more challenging one.
>
> As I explained when we met two days ago, my husband has been transferred to New Orleans and I have been offered a position as occupational health nurse with Ammons and Wilcox Company in the same city. I should like to terminate employment in two weeks although I could arrange to work a bit longer if this will help to orient my replacement.
>
> Again, thank you for your guidance and many kindnesses during the years I have worked at Lawnwood.

The letter opens with a relevant compliment, moves gracefully into the explanation, states the decision after the reasons, and closes positively. The cliché about not burning your bridges behind you applies whenever you have to resign from a position.

SUMMARY

Employment communications are among the most important ones you send as a professional nurse. The six-step job-finding process begins with a self-analysis and market analysis, continues with your résumé and application letter, and concludes with the employment interview and follow-up messages. Communicating about employment in the profession is yet another instance in which the basic principle of adaptation applies.

A necessary first step for entering the job market is a self-analysis or self-appraisal in which you attempt to evaluate yourself from a prospective employer's point of view.

Making a market analysis is the next logical step. Here you research the types of jobs that interest you and the kinds of employers who could use your talents.

Written in outline form, a résumé succinctly yet also specifically lists and discusses your chief qualifications. It is the key document for job seekers and job changers.

When you apply for a position by mail, you send an original application letter together with your résumé. The application letter should be viewed as an informative sales letter that employs the three planned steps of successful selling—attentive interest, desire or conviction, and action ending. Application letters may be solicited (invited) or unsolicited (prospecting).

A special occasion for sharing information and attitudes, the employment interview should be a two-way communication situation between the interviewer and the interviewee. Reviewing the suggestions on what to do before, during, and after an interview can make a difference in how well you succeed in this important face-to-face meeting.

The sixth and last stage in the job-finding process consists of follow-up messages. The thank-you letter, the job acceptance letter, the job refusal letter, and the letter of resignation are the four main types of follow-up messages.

In short, knowledge of and practice in these six communication steps can save you time, give you confidence, and get positive results in the job search.

EXERCISES

1. Make a self-analysis. Prepare a short report of your findings for your instructor, your discussion group, and yourself.
2. Make a market analysis. Prepare a short report of your findings for your instructor, your discussion group, and yourself.
3. Prepare your up-to-date résumé. You may consult examples, but do not copy anyone else's résumé, for that would not do justice to you. Review the guidelines for writing résumés as well as the notes from your self-analysis and market analysis.
4. Prepare an application letter to accompany your résumé. You may apply for a specific position that you have seen advertised or that someone has told you about. Or you may prospect at an agency that may or may not have a vacancy. Review the guidelines and examples in the text. Be sure your letter-résumé package is sendable and accurate.
5. In preparation for future employment interviews, hold mock interviews in class, as your instructor directs. Usually, class members who do not know each other too well exchange letter-résumé packages and

interview each other in turn for about 15 minutes each. When the mock interviews are completed, discuss with the whole class what worked well and what needs to be improved. The experience of someone in your class who has already been out on some interviews might also be worth tapping.

6. Write any two of the four types of follow-up messages discussed in the text. Use specific details, names, and other facts that are based on your experience or projected experience in the job search.

REFERENCES

1. Richard Nelson Bolles, *What Color Is Your Parachute? A Practical Manual for Job-hunters and Career-changers,* 5th ed. (Berkeley, CA: Ten Speed Press, 1978).

2. *Nursing80 Career Directory* (Horsham, PA: Intermed Communications, Inc., 1980).

3. See Herta A. Murphy and Charles E. Peck, *Effective Business Communications,* 3d ed. (New York: McGraw-Hill, 1980), pp. 121–140, for a review of various letter styles.

4. Mary C. Parker, "How to Write Your Resume," *American Journal of Nursing,* 79 (October 1979), 1741.

5. "Career Advice," *Nursing80,* 10 (April 1980), 130.

6. "Make That First Impression Count," in *Nursing79 Career Directory* (Horsham, PA: Intermed Communications, Inc., 1979), p. 30.

7. "Make That First Impression Count," p. 31.

FURTHER READING

Gootnick, David. *Getting a Better Job.* New York: McGraw-Hill, 1978.

Kaiser, Pamela. "Ten Steps to Interviewing Job Applicants." *American Journal of Nursing,* 78 (April 1978), 627–630.

Newcomb, Joan, and Patricia A. Murphy. "The Curriculum Vitae—What It Is and What It Is Not." *Nursing Outlook,* 27 (September 1979), 580–583.

Pearsall, Thomas E., and Donald H. Cunningham. *How to Write for the World of Work.* New York: Holt, Rinehart and Winston, 1978.

Treece, Malra. *Communication for Business and the Professions.* Boston: Allyn and Bacon, 1978.

Walsh, William J. "Preparing a Resume." *American Journal of Nursing,* 74 (April 1974), 677–679.

Wiley, Loy. "Job Interviews: Oh Boy! Are They Important!" *Nursing77,* 7 (August 1977), 65–69.

Wilkinson, C. W., Peter B. Clarke, and Dorothy C. Wilkinson. *Communicating Through Letters and Reports,* 7th ed. Homewood, IL: Irwin, 1980.

Index